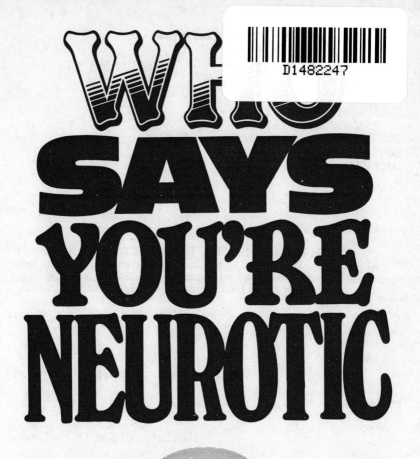

WHO SAYS YOU'RE NEUROTIC

How to Avoid Mistaken
Psychiatric Diagnoses When the Problem
May Be a Physical Condition

Abraham J. Twerski, M.D.

 Prentice-Hall, Inc., Englewood Cliffs, New Jersey 07632

Library of Congress Cataloging in Publication Data

Twerski, Abraham J.
  Who says you're neurotic?

  "A Spectrum Book."
  Includes index.
  1. Mental illness.   I. Title.
RC460.T89 1984   616.89'075   83-27085
ISBN 0-13-958455-2
ISBN 0-13-958448-X (pbk.)

1 2 3 4 5 6 7 8 9 10

ISBN 0-13-958455-2
ISBN 0-13-958448-X {PBK.}

Editorial/production supervision by Peter Jordan
Cover design by Hal Siegel
Manufacturing buyer: Doreen Cavallo

Prentice-Hall International, Inc., *London*
Prentice-Hall of Australia Pty. Limited, *Sydney*
Prentice-Hall Canada Inc., *Toronto*
Prentice-Hall of India Private Limited, *New Delhi*
Prentice-Hall of Japan, Inc., *Tokyo*
Prentice-Hall of Southeast Asia Pte. Ltd., *Singapore*
Whitehall Books Limited, *Wellington, New Zealand*
Editora Prentice-Hall do Brasil Ltda., *Rio de Janeiro*

Contents

Preface

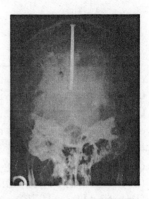

As the dictionary definition points out, the complaint of "I feel I have a nail down the middle of my head" is a hysterical symptom known as *clavus hystericus*. But as the following case demonstrates, this complaint should not be simply dismissed as hysterical.

The skull X-ray shown here is taken from the radiological archives of St. Francis General Hospital, case number 1160-52. The patient in this case was indeed severely mentally ill. She was a psychotic woman who actually took a nail and hammered it through her skull.

Yet this bizarre case does demonstrate the point that just because a symptom corresponds to a classical diagnosis, one should not jump to the conclusion that the diagnosis is correct without fully evaluating the patient and performing an adequate physical examination. There may well be more to the patient's complaints than what appears to be the obvious psychiatric diagnosis.

ABRAHAM J. TWERSKI, M.D., is a practicing psychiatrist. He is clinical director of the Department of Psychiatry at St. Francis General Hospital, Pittsburgh, Pennsylvania, as well as medical director of the Gateway Rehabilitation Center, a treatment facility for alcohol and substance abusers. He is also the author of *Caution: "Kindness" Can Be Dangerous to the Alcoholic* (Prentice-Hall, 1982) and *Like Yourself* *and Others Will Too* (Prentice-Hall, 1978).

Introduction

St. Francis General Hospital in Pittsburgh, with which I have been affiliated since 1965, is a hospital that lends itself particularly well to the analysis of problems in diagnosing mental illnesses.

The psychiatric service at St. Francis comprises more than 200 of the hospital's 700 beds. This unusually large psychiatric component led to the hospital's becoming the emergency and receiving center for psychiatric problems for an area of several million people. For a number of years, more than half of all admissions to the two state hospitals serving the area, with a combined census of 6,000 patients, were funneled through St. Francis for admission evaluation. The combined medical-surgical-psychiatric staff thus had an unusual opportunity to study the complex symptomatology and causes of both psychological and physical illnesses. Many of the cases described in the following pages were processed at St. Francis Hospital.

Although the major portion of this book is concerned with physical illnesses that masquerade as mental problems, it is essential to note that the opposite also occurs—that is, mental illnesses can masquerade as physical illnesses. In either case, failure to make the correct diagnosis precludes effective treatment.

It is also important to recognize that some types of distress signal neither physical nor mental illnesses but are, rather, life situations to which a person must make the most reasonable adjustment feasible. "Therapy" for what is not an illness can be hazardous.

This book is written primarily for the lay public, which has been so widely exposed to mental health problems that many people diagnose themselves as having a psychiatric problem and refer themselves for mental treatment without considering the possibility that they may have a physical disorder. Professionals in the various mental health disciplines may also find this book of value.

Patients, clients, doctors, and therapists are all interested in one common goal: restoring the person to optimum health and functioning. I hope that this book will contribute to that goal.

1

Drunk or Psycho

Martha looked up at the kitchen clock as she heard the front door open and shut. It was 6:20 P.M.

"You could set your clock by Andy's coming home from work," she thought. "Never late. Always comes home directly from the mill and doesn't stop off for 'a shot and a beer' like his friends.

"Andy's a good boy," Martha reflected. Perhaps it wasn't right to think of a grown man of thirty-six as a boy, yet it was difficult not to do so. Martha had helped her sister raise him, and when her sister died, Martha continued to provide a good home for him.

"Supper's on the table, Andy," Martha said. "You'll want to finish early to be on time for the dance. Gail called and said she's expecting you by eight."

Martha had mixed feelings about Andy's relationship with Gail. She certainly had not found fault with her, but, on the other hand, she found herself wishing that Gail and Andy would not marry. She dreaded the thought of the loneliness if Andy were to leave.

Andy came into the kitchen and dropped into a chair. "I don't know about eating, Martha. I haven't felt right all day. My head's been pounding all day long. I stopped off at the dispensary at the mill and got a couple of aspirin, but it seems to have gotten worse. I hate to disappoint Gail, but I don't think I can even make it tonight."

"You're not going to let a headache spoil your evening, Andy," Martha said. "Just eat a little bit, and you'll begin to feel better. It doesn't surprise me, though—your headache, that is. You've been walking around with that chest cold for four weeks, and I've asked you a hundred times to see Dr. McCroy."

Andy took a few teaspoonfuls of gelled fruit, then gently pushed the dish aside. "I don't mean to hurt your feelings, Martha. The food's delicious. It's me that's not right." He arose from the table. "I'm going into a hot shower. Maybe that'll relieve my stiff neck."

Martha cleared the dishes off the table and turned on the television. Some time later Andy came into the living room. "I called Gail and told her I couldn't make it. My head's thumping so bad." Andy stretched out on the reclining chair. "Ouch," he said, "Damn painful neck." Within a few minutes, he was sound asleep.

It was 11:00 o'clock when Martha decided to retire, and Andy was still asleep on the recliner. "No sense in waking him up just to send him to bed," she thought. Martha gently lifted the hair away from Andy's eyes. "He does feel warm," she thought, "I'm going to get this boy to the doctor by hook or crook."

Early the following morning, Martha walked into Andy's room. Andy was sprawled out on his bed, clothes and all. He awoke with a startle as Martha touched his forehead.

"What's the matter, Martha?" Andy asked. He began to sit up in bed. "Oh, my God! Now the pain is all the way down my back," he said. "Can hardly move."

"I'm calling Dr. McCroy," Martha said. "Maybe he can see you right away."

"Forget it, Martha," Andy replied. "It's Saturday morning, and he's not in his office. Anyway, I don't want to go out. Head hurts worse when I move. Just give me some aspirin and I'll be better."

Martha left the room, and returned after a few minutes.

"I talked to Dr. McCroy," she said. "He's on the way to the hospital and said it would be no bother for him to stop off here."

Dr. McCroy was an elderly man. He had delivered Andy and was one of the family. He listened to Andy's chest, checked his throat, and took his blood pressure.

"Nothing that a shot of penicillin won't fix," he said. "Keep up with the aspirin every four hours, and by tomorrow you'll be as good as new."

Andy spent most of the day in bed. He couldn't understand why the aspirin wasn't helping. Dr. McCroy had said he would be feeling better in a day, but by Sunday afternoon, Andy felt worse than ever.

It was about 2:00 A.M. when Martha awoke. She heard the sound of rushing water. She went into the bathroom and both faucets had been fully opened with the water splashing onto the floor. As she went into Andy's room, he sat up in bed and said to her, "Can't come out now. All the trucks and the men at the loading. Oh, my head, dammit! Seventeen trucks. They're all going the other way."

Martha was frightened. "You've had a bad dream, Andy, a nightmare. Let me give you one of my Valiums," she said.

Martha returned to bed and later that morning was awakened by a loud noise. She went down the stairs and there was Andy, pushing the chairs around the dining room. "What are you doing, Andy?" she said.

Andy raised his voice, something he had never done before. "Don't order me around!" he screamed. He pushed the dining room table against the wall, kicked over a chair, then reached for the vase on the table and forcefully threw it at the wall, scattering glass splinters all over the room.

Martha ran back upstairs and dialed the police emergency number. She waited anxiously in her room until she heard the doorbell ring.

When the police arrived, Andy was in the kitchen. Martha

explained to them that her nephew had suddenly begun to act very peculiarly, and she had no idea what brought it on.

"It's simple, lady," the policeman said. "Saturday night, too much booze. Sunday, a hangover. A little bit of the hair of the dog that bit you to fix the hangover, and there you've got it. Where is he?"

Martha showed the police officers into the kitchen. Andy was sitting on the floor. The refrigerator door was open, and all of the contents of the refrigerator had been placed on the kitchen floor. Andy looked up at the police officers with bewilderment.

"Too much boozing, eh, buddy?" the officer remarked. "You're scaring the old lady with your antics. Get up now and get back into bed where you can sleep it off."

"But Andy doesn't drink," Martha protested. "This isn't like him."

The officer laughed. "Don't let him fool you. None of 'em drink, lady, they just guzzle." The officers reached down to help Andy to his feet, but as he was getting up, Andy pushed at one officer and kicked the other. "So that's how it's going to be, eh?" one of the officers said. Within moments, a struggling and screaming Andy was being escorted into the police wagon.

"Take him to Memorial Hospital," Martha cried. "It's just down the block, and Dr. McCroy is his doctor! There's something wrong with the boy!"

"Relax, lady," the officers told her. "Your boy will be okay. We get these guys every weekend. Climb in the front seat and come along. We'll take him where he'll get help."

The police wagon raced down the street, lights, flashing and siren blaring. As they passed Memorial Hospital, one of the officers said, "No point in taking a drunk to Memorial, lady. They don't like drunks there, especially a wild one like this. Only place to go is St. Francis."

"But I'm telling you, Andy doesn't drink," Martha insisted.

"Well, if that's the case, then he's gone psycho, and then he really belongs in St. Francis," the officer replied.

The doctor on call was reviewing some records at his desk when Sister Margaret interrupted. "There are some police out here with a patient. I told them to go to the emergency room, but they said he's for psychiatry."

The doctor went to the admissions office, where he found the two police officers trying to restrain a wildly thrashing, screaming man, who looked for all the world like a drunk in DTs. "Here's one for you, doc. He's either boozing too much or he's gone psycho."

The lady accompanying the police said, "That's not true! Andy doesn't drink." She then related to the doctor the events of the past two days, with the abrupt change in Andy's behavior.

"Where do we take him to, doc?" the police asked. "We've got him here, and we have to get going back."

"Hold it a minute, guys," the doctor said. He turned to Martha. "Look, ma'am, if Andy has not been drinking, then there is trouble here. We need you to sign a permit for a spinal tap."

"Never!" Martha said. "I know of a woman who had a spinal tap and never walked again."

"Well, then you will have to take him back home with you," the doctor said. "I can hardly treat a patient if I don't have the ability to do the necessary examination and tests."

Reluctantly, Martha signed the authorization, and the police, with the help of several nursing assistants, carried Andy into the psychiatric unit.

A little later that day, the director of the laboratory called the admitting physcian.

"The spinal tap shows meningitis. The spinal fluid is full of pus. Better get the patient into isolation quickly," he said. Within moments, the intravenous fluids were carrying life-saving antibiotics into Andy's veins.

Andy recovered from a severe meningoencephalitis, an infection affecting the brain and spinal cord, and his "craziness" disappeared completely. A more thorough examination revealed a tiny sinus, or a little opening in Andy's back. Investigation of this revealed that Andy had had an abscess that had formed a sinus tract that had perforated his back muscles, went through the right kidney, dissected behind the liver and through the diaphragm, went through the right lung and into the right bronchus. Andy had been harboring a chronic infection that had spread to the brain, and this had produced the mental symptoms.

The police wagon had passed up the hospital just two blocks from Andy's home, where his personal physician was on the staff. They also passed three other general hospitals enroute to St. Francis, because Andy was obviously mentally ill. He was either "drunk or psycho."

Anyone looking at Andy would probably have concurred with the police officer's diagnosis. But if Andy had been assumed to be "psycho" for another twenty-four hours, he would have died.

2

Problems in
the Diagnosis
of Mental Illness

Whereas the incidence of erroneous diagnosis of florid psychoses, which are in reality a manifestation of physical disorders, may be low, this is of little comfort to the patient so misdiagnosed or to the family who must adjust to the consequences of a diagnosis of serious mental illness. In the case of diagnoses of neuroses or of other emotional disorders, the incidence of error is not at all negligible.

In one study involving more than 2,000 patients referred to a psychiatric clinic, 43 percent of the patients had major medical illnesses, and close to half of those had not been diagnosed by the referring service. Of those patients, 32 percent referred by various physicians had undiagnosed major physical illnesses. Of those referred by psychiatrists, 42 percent had major medical diagnoses that had been missed. Of patients who were self-referred or referred by social agencies, *more than 80 percent* had an undiagnosed major medical illness. In 69 percent of the cases, the undiagnosed medical illness contributed considerably to the psychiatric symptoms. In one out of five cases, the physical illness alone was responsible for the psychiatric problem.[1]

Even when a patient is medically evaluated, physical dis-

[1]E. K. Koranyi, "Morbidity and Role of Undiagnosed Physical Illnesses in Psychiatric Clinic Population," *Archives of General Psychiatry* 36 (April 1979): 414–419; Koranyi, "Undiagnosed Physical Illness in Psychiatric Patients," *Annual Review of Medicine* 33 (1982): 309–396.

orders may go undetected if the physician's index of suspicion is not sufficiently high. Articles in the medical literature call attention to possible physical origins of many "mental" diseases, but too often these go unheeded.[2]

There is yet another pitfall in the diagnosis of mental or emotional illness and that is "diagnosis by exclusion." If a patient persists in complaining of some discomfort after all diagnostic tests have failed to reveal any physical disorder, the doctor is too often apt to say "your problem is psychosomatic," "it's all in your imagination," or something that carries the same connotation.

Diagnosis by exclusion is very poor medicine. First, it assumes that the doctor, or for that matter medical science, knows all there is to know about the human body in health and disease, and this is simply not true. For all that we do know about human physiology and biochemistry, the honest physician will admit that what is not known exceeds that which is known. The counterpart of today's omniscient physician 30 years ago was equally certain of his omniscience yet might not have imagined that there would be new techniques to permit detailed and accurate visualization of internal structures, or tests that could confirm or eliminate certain diagnoses with a high degree of accuracy. Similarly, techniques 30 years hence will demonstate how relatively limited our current medical knowledge is.

Truly honest physicians are humble people, humbled by their awareness of how much they do not and cannot know at a particular stage of medical science. To these physicians, the accumulation of negative findings leads only to the conclusion

[2]R. H. Culpan, B. M. Davis, and A. N. Oppenheim, "Incidence of Psychiatric Illness Among Hospital Outpatients," *British Medical Journal* 19: (1960) 855–857; W. D. Davies, "Physical Illness in Psychiatric Outpatients," *British Journal of Psychiatry* 111 (1965): 27–37; G. P. Maguire, and K. L. Granville-Grossman "Physical Illness in Psychiatric Patients," *British Medical Journal* 115 (1968): 1365–1369; R. C. W. Hall, M. D. Popkin, R. DeVaul, L. A. Faillace, and S. K. Stickney, "Physical Illness Presenting as Psychiatric Disease," *Archives of General Psychiatry* 35 (1978): 11, 1315–1320.

of "I don't know what is causing your discomfort" and nothing else.

Second, just as with any other diagnosis, a psychiatric diagnosis must be supported by evidence. There are indeed grounds for making the diagnosis of a mental or emotional disorder. When these criteria are met, such a diagnosis is justified but not otherwise.

I once received a patient on the psychiatric service who was transferred from the surgical service with a diagnosis of "psychogenic pain." This patient had been complaining of vague abdominal distress. I called the surgeon, who advised me that he considered the patient neurotic because all the X-rays had failed to show any organic pathology.

This disturbed me a great deal. To make my point, I returned the patient to the surgical service with a diagnosis of "cancer of the tail of the pancreas," a condition that cannot be diagnosed without exploratory surgery. The surgeon called me and asked me on what grounds I had made this diagnosis, and I responded that inasmuch as I could not discover any emotional problem, the pain was undoubtedly caused by cancer of the tail of the pancreas. I pointed out to him that his psychiatric diagnosis had no greater validity than my physical diagnosis. Only then did the surgeon realize how unsound it was to make a positive diagnosis on the basis of absence of evidence.

A combined medical-surgical-psychiatric case conference was then arranged. Social service staff provided invaluable insights into some of the environmental problems affecting the patient. Although the conference did not yield an absolute diagnosis, all those attending had a comprehensive understanding of the patient. The patient was then advised that the source of his pain was not clear and that ongoing contact with both the surgical and psychiatric departments was recommended.

Depressive illnesses may have some physical discomfort or physical dysfunction as their primary presenting symptoms. But depression is a condition with many features, and there are criteria for making a diagnosis of depression. There is no justification, however, for assuming that the problem must be depression just because a patient has no evident physical abnormalities. Not infrequently some definite physical illness makes itself known only after a period of time. If the patient is simply sloughed off as being "psycho," the proper follow-up may not be provided, and an otherwise treatable illness may be allowed to progress.

The interdisciplinary team approach, with input from experts in psychiatry, internal medicine, psychology, social service, nursing, and rehabilitation, offers the best method for avoiding a mistaken diagnosis. Unfortunately, the ideal of team approach is not always achieved.

The mind–body dichotomy that was inherited from previous eras has not yet been overcome by a more holistic philosophy. Consequently, some mental health clinics, designed to provide easier access to mental health services, lack adequate medical participation in evaluation of patients who have primarily emotional disorders. Similarly, physicians trained to approach a human being as a conglomerate of organs or organ systems may be unaware that feelings do not exist in some void separate from the body but are an integral part of the person. Until such fragmentation is overcome, serious diagnostic errors are apt to occur.

3

Depression

Although some people may think that seeing a psychiatrist is a status symbol, many people resent being told that they should consult a psychiatrist. Emotional problems and mental illness are still often stigmatized. This stigma may be a residual of the ancient belief that these conditions were evil and caused by demoniacal possession, or it may be because of the assumption that emotional and mental problems are a result of moral degeneration or character weaknesses. One still often hears relatives tell a patient to "just make up his mind" or "take hold of himself and pull himself together." In cases of *bona fide* depression, this is adding insult to injury. Depressed people want nothing more than to pull themselves out of their misery.

According to the dualistic mind–body concept, the body was considered to be legitimately subject to trauma, infection, and metabolic disorders, but the mind was supposed to be some ethereal entity, removed from all physical accidents and completely under domination of the will. Hence, any dysfunction of the mind is apt to be considered an indication that one must be weak-willed.

Because physical illnesses can often be documented by tissue changes, by blood test abnormalities, or on X-ray, people assume that diseases cause these conditions. But because emotional disorders often do not have any tangible laboratory abnormality, emotional conditions are often not considered "genuine" diseases.

The phenomena of depression lend themselves quite readily to psychological explanations. Doctors have long known that the majority of depressive patients feel their worst in the early morning and tend to improve later on during the day. This sequence had been explained as being caused by the people's frustration on arising and realizing that they must push through another full day of misery; whereas when the night approaches, the promise of escape from the torment during sleep provides a modicum of relief. Postpartum depressions were understood as a reaction to the "loss" of the pregnancy, and postmenopausal depression was considered a reaction to the woman's perception of the loss of her youth. The paramenstrual "blues" were explained as the woman's unconscious resentment of her femininity or her disappointment at not being pregnant. The latter explanation was considered valid even for a woman for whom pregnancy would have been a total disaster. In his classic work *Mourning and Melancholia*, Freud compares depression to grief and demonstrates how and why the grief reaction to a loss remains within normal range and how and why the depressive reaction, which is assumed to always be a response to a loss, results in a pathological state. When everything was understood to be on a purely psychological basis, treatment for these conditions was assumed to be essentially of a psychological nature.

These theories came under serious scrutiny in the 1950s. Several years earlier, a derivative from the rawolfia plant, which had been used in India for many years, was introduced into the Western world for treatment of high blood pressure and also as a major tranquilizer. After the medication was in widespread use, doctors noted that a small percentage of patients who were treated with rawolfia developed severe depressions, identical in every way to a classical depressive psychosis, even including suicide. Treatment of these depressions often required nothing more than simply discontinuing the medication, following which the patient's mood gradually returned to normal. Here, then, were instances where nothing of significance had changed in the patient's life. All variables were constant except for a chemical change in the body as a result of medication. It became apparent that at least some depressions were of chemical rather than psychological origin.

An experience that occurred during my psychiatric residency further influenced my personal orientation. Having suffered with hayfever for many years, I was prescribed a new potent decongestant medication. Shortly after I began taking this medication, I began to notice I was losing interest in things and had difficulty concentrating. I had no interest in what I read, and I could not retain the information. Soon thereafter I lost my appetite, and all food seemed to taste like cardboard. I was aware that something was amiss, yet I delayed consulting one of my instructors in psychiatry. Then I began awakening at 2:00 A.M., feeling agitated, trapped and doomed to be this way forever. Life began to appear burdensome; in the early hours of the morning, I decided that on the following day I would seek psychiatric help.

The following day at breakfast I was about to take my hayfever medication when it suddenly occurred to me that the change of mood I had been experiencing coincided with the use of this medication. I therefore discontinued the medication and had a prompt return of the hayfever symptoms—but within several days the depression completely disappeared. Several months later, I came across several reports in the medical literature relating depression to decongestant medication. The chemical etiology of my depression was thus firmly established.

In the 1960s, refined techniques of measuring the neurohormones that circulate in the body provided some evidence that biochemical changes occur in the depressed patient, and we now have adequate grounds to assume that in many of the severe depressive syndromes, chemical changes are causative.[1] In addition to causes of a purely psychological nature, these

---

[1]G. Winokur, *Depression, the Facts.* (London: Oxford University Press, 1981), 86–99.

changes may also occur after anything that upsets the body physiology, such as menopause, childbirth, surgery of any type, hepatitis, premenstruum, or even as an aftermath of a common virus. Changes may occur after exhaustion, such as after prolonged sleeplessness. They can also occur without an apparent precipitating cause. Considerable evidence shows that these chemical changes are familial and have a genetic pattern. They may occur irregularly or in some cyclical pattern, such as every spring or every eighteen months. They may also alternate with episodes of euphoria and increased activity.

Some investigators have presented evidence that in the depressed patient, the neurohormones that are involved are at their lowest level in the early morning hours and rise slowly toward a daily maximum in the evening. Hence, the explanation of the daily fluctuations of the mood of the depressed patient is one of a chemical nature rather than being purely psychological, as was earlier assumed.

In those cases of depression that are biochemical, therapy that consists solely of searching for the psychological cause is not going to be productive. However, as mentioned earlier, two intimate people cannot interact without having some areas of conflict, and if one looks only for psychological conflicts in the depressed patient, one will find them. Indeed, if one looks for psychological conflict in the *non*depressed person, one will find it there, too. It is simple to ascribe the depressed patient's symptoms to these conflicts and even to counsel separation from family members or divorce as a solution. Such manuevers frequently are tragic, because not only do they not address the true origin of the illness, but they also may intensify areas of conflict that may actually be insignificant in the person's life and may generate strife where none existed. Separation and divorce may also deprive the depressed patient of major and meaningful sources of love and support.

Depressed people's pathological moods may be likened to looking at the world through dark glasses or distorting lenses.

Their perceptions of reality may thus not be factual. The hostility they express toward others or that they feel others have toward them may be artifacts of the mood disorder; it is hazardous to take these feelings at their face value.

The initial treatment of those conditions that are primarily biochemical in origin is essentially chemical—the body's chemical imbalance is corrected by using the appropriate medications and occasionally by electrical stimulation. Initial psychotherapy in these cases should generally not be of the searching, uncovering, and insight-oriented type, but rather supportive—that is to help the patient through the rough period until the effective medications are found that will correct the condition. After the pathological mood has been corrected, the doctor must evaluate possible psychological causes or contributing factors to the depression. Time is on the patient's side, because depressive episodes always run their course and eventually remit even without treatment. However, treatment is essential because it is simply inhumane to allow a long siege of depression to continue, and sometimes the depression can be so severe that the patient attempts suicide.

Thus, people need to recognize that although the symptoms of depression are "mental," the mechanism of the condition is often physical. Just as some physical changes can result in respiratory diseases, blood diseases, or digestive tract diseases, these particular physical changes result in diseases or dysfunction of the thinking–feeling systems. It is grossly incorrect to assume that depressed patients truly resent or hate their spouse, children, siblings, and parents. The bitterness that occurs during depression is no more a reflection of the people's true feelings than would be any feeling or verbalization expressed while they were in a delirium with a fever of one hundred and six degrees. Treatment of the depressed patient requires expert consideration of the totality of the patient, physical as well as social and psychological, and appropriate institution of the correct treatment at the right time.

While people with asthma or arthritis bewail their condition (why me?), they generally do not go about feeling guilty about their misery. On the other hand, depressives not only suffer intensely but also feel profound guilt for being depressed, as if they were depressed by choice. Very often depressives will say, "Why am I doing this to myself?" Depressed patients and their families must be helped to realize that the disease is of a physical, biological character, and that guilt has no justification.

A frequent behavioral upset that is primarily of biochemical origin is the premenstrual syndrome. This is a commonly occurring condition that has not received its due in the medical literature and whose importance has been more publicized by the lay media.

People have known since time immemorial that shortly before the menstrual period many women tend to be "out of sorts," with various symptoms such as headache, cramping, swelling of the fingers and ankles, and irritability. Many women simply adjust to the few unpleasant days, and some obtain relief with mild medication.

What has not been appreciated is that the premenstrual symptoms may last for half of the month and may be intense, thus actually prevailing over half of the adult woman's life. Women also have a carryover from the "sick" half month to the "well" half month, so that the majority of the women's lives can be spent in misery. Furthermore, rather than having symptoms of merely annoying character, women may become extremely depressed and even suicidal during this phase, may turn to alcohol and initiate an alcoholism or chemical–dependency problem, or may abuse their children.[2]

The depressed feelings in the premenstrual syndrome may be indistinguishable from those seen in major depressive dis-

---

[2] K. Dalton, *The Premenstrual Syndrome and Progesterone Therapy*, (Chicago: Year Book Publisher, 1977), 36; Z. R. Graves, and N. H. Lauersen, M.D., "A New Approach to Premenstrual Syndrome," *The Female Patient*, Vol. 8, April 1983.

orders. Women may exhibit agitation or lethargy, bitterness, resentment, and self-denigration. The woman may manifest
extreme hostility toward her husband, children, parents, and
other family members. Serious family arguments may occur.
Frustrations with the children may result in harsh beatings.

Although the chemical changes resolve after several days
and the woman's mood returns to normal, the acrimonious remarks and hostile expressions cannot be easily retracted. These
have made their impact and tend to leave scars, if not open
wounds. The woman may have had some preexisting difficulties
with the in-laws to which she has adjusted and which could
have ultimately been resolved. But, if during a premenstrual
depression, she becomes hyperirritable and denounces them for
their meddling or overpossessiveness and orders them out of
her house never to return, those words are not easily retracted
nor forgotten and may cause a rift between husband and wife.
The couple may have had some differences between them, but
if the wife's hostility is intensified during the premenstruum
and she explodes with violent criticism of her husband, the
hostlity is not easily undone. The woman may refuse to have
sex with her husband during the depressed phase, and he may
take this as a personal rejection rather than a manifestation of
his wife's depression. If the woman was abusive toward the
children, she may be guilt-laden after the premenstruum. Thus,
very destructive aftereffects can prevent restoration of normal
mood after the hormonal changes restabilize.

If the problems are severe enough to warrant seeking professional help and the nature of the premenstrual syndrome is
not recognized, the therapist may focus on the areas of conflict
between the couple or between family members. Too often the
resurrection of differences that had essentially been resolved
can have the opposite effect of re-igniting or exaggerating interpersonal conflicts rather than eliminating them. These may
again emerge in a subsequent premenstrual phase and can result
in severe deterioration of relationships.

The laity and the medical and psychological professions need to be more aware of the role of the premenstrual syndrome. Just the recognition that in some cases the woman is truly "not herself" can be helpful. Even in the absence of any treatment, the husband should realize that he must discount some things the wife says at this time and must not respond to them as if they were indications of her true feelings. He can be very helpful if he is particularly sensitive to her needs at this time and if he gives some assistance with the care of the children. The in-laws should similarly adjust in a manner wherein they recognize that the woman's behavior is alien to her. Although these adjustments may not alter the woman's mood, they can eliminate aggravation of the condition and prevent the carryover to the postmenstrual phase.

Some medical interventions can help in cases of severe symptoms, but the application of such treatment presupposes recognition of the condition.[3] Unless there is such recognition, the woman with a serious premenstrual syndrome who consults a psychiatrist for depression and whose marriage may have been seriously affected as described above may be misdiagnosed and may end up with inappropriate psychotherapy and chemotherapy.

A twenty-five-year-old mother of two was referred for psychiatric treatment because of recurrent depression. The young woman appeared desperate and reported that she could not see how she could go on much longer. She stated that shortly after the birth of her first child, she began to suffer recurrent depressions. These were characterized by complete inability to do anything—she would simply lie in bed all day, unable even to eat. She would cry, would fly into fits of rage at her husband and anyone else around, and felt herself to be unsafe with her her children. She had more than once contemplated suicide,

[3]Dalton, *The Premenstrual Syndrome and Progesterone Therapy* 73–83; R. V. Norris, and Sullivan, *PMS—Premenstrual Syndrome* (New York: Ramson Associates, 1983), 187–256.

although she had never actually made an attempt. During the depressive episodes, she would have the children cared for by her friends because she could not attend to their needs because she was afraid she might harm them.

The patient had been prescribed various antidepressants but said that these had actually made her symptoms worse.

The young woman said she could not understand why she was so depressed because in the intervals between depressions she was happy, enthusiastic, and a devoted wife and mother. She loved to be with people and do creative things around the house. There was no indication that these intervals were euphoric or related to any manic episodes. However, when the depression struck, she became totally incapacitated. "It's like being two different people," she said. "I become a monster. I don't even know myself. When I am in one of these, everything looks hopeless. You can't even talk to me, because I just can't understand what you're saying." The husband corroborated her account.

As the woman described the pattern of her depressions, it became evident that they were related to her menses. Approximately ten days before her period was due, the depression would start abruptly. The depression would end just as quickly on the second or third day of the next cycle. Doctors felt that this woman had a classic premenstrual syndrome, and because of the severity of the symptoms, she was prescribed progesterone in suppository form. The very first course of treatment produced total relief from all the depressive symptoms.

Contrary to popular opinion, the premenstrual syndrome can occur after menopause and even after a hysterectomy. Women who may not have had premenstrual problems may develop serious emotional symptoms during or after the menopause.

During the menopause a woman's physiology undergoes a major overhaul. Many women are bothered with distressing hot flashes and sweating, which are sometimes followed by chills.

That these symptoms have been related to hormonal changes has been widely recognized. However, when the woman develops crying spells, dejection, loss of appetite, loss of interest, loss of sexual desire, and agitation or lethargy, we for some reason implicate psychological factors such as loss of youth or desertion by her children, who are at this time generally becoming independent. While these are certainly important emotional considerations, they are frequently not primary in causing the depression. Rather, proper medication often relieves the symptoms and returns the woman to normal mood, although the lost youth has not returned and the empty nest is still empty. Once the woman has been successfully treated for her depression, she can generally adjust to this new phase of her life.

As with the premenstrual syndrome, the negative behaviors that emerge in the menopausal depression can be disruptive unless they are understood to be manifestations of a distorted body chemistry. Furthermore, people are much more apt to seek medical help with physical than with psychological problems, probably because they believe that they should be able to master the latter on their own. Being aware that these conditions are also of physical rather than purely psychological or characterological origin should make it easier for the woman to seek help. And those in her environment are more likely to be empathetic with a person who is a victim of a physical–chemical disease than they would be with one who is a frustrated, bitter person who is unappreciative of her family.

One of the most frequent symptoms of depression is fatigue. Along with feeling dejected, a person is apt to have lassitude and a total lack of energy, which may be interpreted by both patient and therapist as a loss of interest.

Many physical conditions may bring about fatigue, lassitude, and loss of interest, and a thorough medical evaluation may often reveal the source of the problem. If it is assumed from the outset, however, that the problem is purely a psychological one, the true state of affairs may go undiscovered.

A common cause of persistent fatigue is anemia. Anemia can be the result of poor nutrition, which is not at all limited to poverty. Some well-to-do people have poor dietary habits, and if they use alcohol to any degree, they are quite apt to be anemic. People may have chronic blood loss, as from a slowly bleeding peptic ulcer that may be painless or from regular use of aspirin as with chronic arthritis. They may have a hereditary hemoglobin disease, a chronic low-grade infection, or lymphocytic leukemia. Conditions such as these sometimes do not produce any other symptom that would direct the patient's attention to consult a physician, and the only symptoms may be fatigue, lassitude, and depression.

Claudia was a seventeen-year-old high school senior who could have been the prototype of the "student most likely to succeed." She had always achieved good grades, was well liked by her teachers and classmates, and was very active in extracurricular activities. She had been elected president of her class and was in competition to become valedictorian. She appeared to be well-adjusted at home, and she had not shown any indication of emotional instability.

One night on the way home from a date, the car Claudia was in was involved in an accident. Claudia was rendered unconscious momentarily, but except for minor cuts from bits of broken glass, neither she nor her boyfriend were seriously injured. She was evaluated briefly in a hospital emergency room and released.

Within several weeks after the accident, Claudia began having severe headaches. Her physician referred her to a neurologist, and a thorough evaluation, including a CAT scan of the brain and an electroencephalogram, showed no sign of physical damage to the head.[4] All her blood studies were normal. The doctor found no indication for any specific treatment, and

[4]The CAT (Computerized Axial Tomography) scan is a radiologic study which provides a precise analysis of the brain, just as if the physician were able to examine the brain layer by layer. This is accomplished without anything being done to the brain itself and is thus a very safe and revealing diagnostic method.

Claudia found that she obtained some degree of relief from aspirin.

Claudia was at this time in a highly stressful situation. She carried on with her functions as class president and with her various activities and studied diligently to maintain her grade-point average. She did this in spite of persistent and fairly constant headaches, for which she reverted to repeated doses of aspirin. Within a very short time, Claudia was taking 12 to 15 aspirins daily.

About four months after the accident, Claudia began to experience progressive fatigue. She was unable to get up early in the morning, and her sleep pattern was irregular. She became irritable with the family, and her scholastic performance deteriorated. The headaches continued unabated.

Inasmuch as the neurological examination had been negative, Claudia's difficulties were assumed to be emotional, and she consulted a psychologist. Psychological evaluation revealed Claudia to be an overachiever to whom success was all-important. Claudia had some unwarranted feelings of inferiority, from which she sought relief by attaining scholastic excellence, a position of leadership, and the expression of esteem by her peers.

Nothing was fundamentally wrong with Claudia's adjustment, but the automobile accident had seriously interfered with her way of life. No doubt, the trauma of the accident had precipitated some emotional difficulty, and the headaches that followed set up a serious vicious cycle. Claudia's successful adjustment had been achieved by her diligence and by expending a great deal of energy in study and in her social activities; the recurrent headaches detracted from her performance. As she felt her ability to achieve her goals as valedictorian and class leadership threatened by the disabling headaches, she became increasingly tense and anxious. The tension and anxiety further intensified the headaches, so that a self-reinforcing and self-perpetuating vicious cycle had begun.

All of these psychological conclusions were without doubt correct, and Claudia was seen regularly by the psychologist, who did his utmost to reduce the anxiety and help her accept herself as worthwhile even if she were not to succeed in becoming "number one." However, in spite of excellent psychotherapy, Claudia's condition deteriorated.

Claudia then missed two menstrual periods, and although this is not an unusual occurrence in a young woman in a highly stressful situation, she consulted a gynecologist. In the process of this evaluation, her blood count revealed a severe anemia with a hemoglobin of 7 gm%, or about fifty percent of normal. Evaluation of the anemia revealed the culprit to be the large amount of aspirin Claudia had been taking for her headaches. These had irritated the lining of her stomach, resulting in slow but steady bleeding. There had not been any sudden hemorrhage to call attention to blood loss, and but for the blood test ordered by the gynecologist, the anemia could have remained undetected.

In Claudia's case, the help that the psychotherapy was providing was counteracted by the lassitude, weakness, and exhaustion resulting from the anemia. As the latter drained Claudia's energies, her anxiety over her inability to achieve was intensified, and the anemia initiated another vicious cycle.

The use of aspirin is so widespread that few people think of it as a potentially dangerous drug. Claudia certainly did not think it worthwhile to bring to anyone's attention, and the psychologist had good reason to feel reassured that the fairly recent medical workup had eliminated any physical cause for Claudia's emotional difficulties, as indeed it had at the time. Particularly in an era when over-the-counter medications are widely used, periodic physical reevaluation should be considered with any prolonged emotional problem.

Malignancies may have depression as their first symptom. Cancer of the pancreas is particularly known to often be manifested first by depression; in such instances, time is crucial, because the chance of effective medical or surgical treatment can be lost by delay.

Hepatitis does not always produce the tell-tale sign of jaundice. The patient with viral hepatitis or with liver disease from infectious mononucleosis may have a fever and other symptoms characteristic of the "flu" and may not seek medical attention for this. He may subsequently develop a classic depression with fatigue, loss of appetite, and lassitude as prominent features. With nothing striking to call attention to the liver as the involved organ, the patient may be treated psychotherapeutically for what is assumed to be a psychogenic depession.

I wish to reemphasize a point made earlier. Things in every person's life can be grounds for dissatisfaction. Many people have financial difficulties. Their jobs may be frustrating. Perhaps their work is boring and unchallenging, or perhaps their bosses make unrealistic demands. People may be dissatisfied with their living arrangements and may be in situations where they cannot make a change. Children are frequently a source of concern. They may not be doing well in school or may have social problems; or they may be smoking marijuana or be defiant of their parents. There are many things in people's lives that they would certainly prefer to be different.

If the therapist evaluating a depressed patient discovers some obvious source of discontent in the person's life, the therapist may attribute the depression to these factors, and treatment may then focus on these. In those instances where the depression is largely a consequence of a physical problem, the wrong conclusion may lead to a medical problem going untreated.

More information about the Premenstrual Syndrome can be obtained from:

Premenstrual Syndrome Action, Inc.
P.O. Box 9326
Madison, WI 53715 *or*
The National PMS Society
P.O. Box 11467
Durham, NC 27703

4

Anxiety

Anxiety is a most distressing symptom and one that frequently motivates people to seek psychological or psychiatric therapy.

What is anxiety? Suppose you are driving down a steep hill on a winter day and suddenly find the road to be so icy and slippery that you have no control of your car. Stepping on the brakes does no good, and the car does not respond to your efforts to steer. Down ahead, at the bottom of the hill, the road intersects with a busy thoroughfare. You know for certain that you are going to be hit by an oncoming car and be seriously maimed or killed. You are helpless to do anything to avert the inevitable disaster. If you somehow escape being hit, you may subsequently recall that you had felt a sense of impending doom. You may recall that your throat constricted, you felt a choking sensation, you gasped for air, and you felt your heart fluttering. You may have screamed or may have felt too paralyzed with fear to scream. You knew something horrible was going to happen to you and were totally unable to do anything to escape your doom.

Such a situation is not difficult to imagine, and one can certainly empathize with the victim of such circumstances. That person's feelings are those of intense fear.

Suppose that the exact same sensations occur not in a situation of actual danger, but when you are standing in the checkout line of a supermarket, or driving along level terrain on a clear sunny day, or sitting quietly at church services. Suddenly, out of nowhere, you are seized by a paroxysm of intense fear, with the identical feelings described above: palpitation, constriction of the throat, air hunger, tremors, and a sense of impending doom. You might wish to scream, but you hold back because you don't want to appear stupid. You would like to run for your life, but you don't want to create an embarrassing scene, or perhaps your legs feel so wooden that you can't even move them. Whereas these feelings were certainly appropriate while skidding down an icy slope, they are most inappropriate when you are in a quiet, nonthreatening setting. The latter is what is referred to as anxiety; it is a distressing sensation and one that is incomprehensible to the individual because nothing immediate warrants such intense fear.

Sigmund Freud, who so beautifully described the workings of the unconscious mind, postulated that fear and anxiety are essentially identical; that is, they are both reactions to a devastating threat. The only difference is that in the case of fear, the threat is evident and obvious to the subject and often to outside observers; in the case of anxiety, the threat is hidden not only from others, but even from the subject himself. The danger is perceived by the subject's *unconscious* mind, hence he has no awareness of it.

Freud said that many thoughts and feelings exist in the unconscious mind, and they may elicit a reaction just as or even more intense than a conscious idea. For example, a man is in the company of someone he loves dearly and has a severe anxiety attack. Freud says that he may have an urge or impulse of which he was unaware to do something harmful to this person whom he loves. Or while sitting in church, he has an urge or impulse, of which he is unaware, to scream out an obscenity or expose himself, which would have an utterly devastating effect on his social standing. Such urges and impulses constitute real threats or dangers to the individual, and his system reacts to them just as though they were objective dangers. Inasmuch as the subject is not aware of them, the anxiety response is incomprehensible to him.

The symptoms listed earlier that generally accompany fear or anxiety are those of the "fight or flight" response; that is, when people are confronted by a danger, they have only one of two possible options: to fight the threatening object or to run away from it. To either attack or escape, the body mobilizes itself by a number of physiologic changes that maximize the capacity to attack or escape. The heart rate increases to pump more blood to energize the muscles, and the blood supply is shifted from the digestive organs to the muscles. Breathing is accelerated to bring more oxygen into the system. Some muscles may go into spasm as the body becomes rigid. The pupils dilate to maximize vision, and the liver pours blood sugar into the circulation to supply the requisite energy for the encounter. All of these are adaptations of the body to coping with a threat and are mediated by various chemicals in the body, the best known of which is adrenalin.

In the case of fear, where the source of danger is known and evident, people can attempt to either overcome the threat or escape. Neither of those options is possible in the case of anxiety, because the source of danger is perceived only by the unconscious mind, and the subject is not aware of what it is that he must master or flee. Hence, fear generally has an end point, while anxiety may be of indefinite duration.

Another difficulty with anxiety is that it is apt to be self-reinforcing. For example, a student who is faced with an important exam and who has a good grasp of the material to be covered by the exam may become anxious when actually confronted with the exam. Perhaps so much of his self-esteem is at stake that the possibility of doing poorly on the exam is a severe threat. The symptoms of anxiety may become so distressing that they impair his ability to concentrate and recall. As he becomes aware of his difficulty in recalling the subject material, he becomes even more fearful that he will fail, and this then generates more anxiety, which further impairs his thinking ability. Thus you have a vicious cycle, and one that is not an infrequent reason that good students may do poorly on exams. In many instances of anxiety, a vicious cycle is set in motion that feeds upon itself until it becomes a panic reaction.

The self-reinforcing, self-perpetuating vicious cycle phenomenon is crucial to understanding anxiety. Because anxiety begets anxiety, it becomes cause as well as effect. This holds true regardless of what initiates the anxiety. Thus, if the body were to receive jolts of adrenalin or other stimulating chemicals from any source, the resultant symptoms could generate new anxiety. Furthermore, anxiety attacks can be so distressful that the anticipation of an attack may be an adequate stimulus to bring on an attack.

Freud's formulation holds true for many cases of anxiety. It is less certain his theory explains all cases.

Just as an example, a very rare disease causes classic anxiety symptoms and is caused by excessive production and release of adrenalin by a tumor of the adrenal gland (pheochromocytoma). In contrast to the common type of anxiety attack where the emotional reaction brings about the release of adrenalin, the reverse occurs in pheocromocytoma, with the release of adrenalin causing the anxiety reaction.

Pheochromocytoma is rare and so has nothing to do with most cases of anxiety. But the point that it demonstrates is that a physical change *can* bring about the emotional reaction instead of the reverse. Because of the vicious cycle and anticipation phenomena, anxiety attacks that may have been physically initiated may acquire an independent existence.

Physical changes that can result in anxiety symptoms may occur in several ways. Some medications contain stimulants that mimic the actions of adrenalin, such as decongestants or bronchodialators prescribed for sinus congestion or asthma, respectively; these drugs are commonly available even without a prescription. Diet pills have a similar action, and caffeine has also been implicated in anxiety. On the other hand, discontinuing some medications that the person has been using regularly may produce anxiety symptoms as part of the withdrawal reaction.

Coronary artery disease may be mistaken for an anxiety attack. Hyperthyroidism has many of the features of anxiety. In all, about fifty physical problems, some rare and some not so rare, can result in anxiety.[1]

Anxiety attacks caused by drug reactions or other physical causes may be self-limited and usually disappear when the underlying cause is eliminated. However, because of the tendency of anxiety to self-perpetuate, attacks may persist even after the initiating cause is no longer operative. The longer the attacks persist, the more apt the condition is to become chronic. Hence, early identification of physical causes of anxiety is of utmost importance.

[1]R. C. W. Hall, *Psychiatric Presentations of Medical Illness* (New York: Spectrum Publishers, 1980), 13–35.

5

Hyperventilation

Hyperventilation frequently occurs as one of the many symptoms of anxiety. It warrants particular attention because it can lead to other symptoms that may be mistaken for more serious illness or psychoses.

As the term implies, hyperventilation refers to an increase in breathing. Some people with anxiety episodes describe a feeling of "air hunger" and are aware that they felt unable to breathe deeply and that they were breathing rapidly and shallowly. Some describe a suffocating sensation, sometimes accompanied by chest pain, and recall feeling as though they were having a heart attack. They often feel that if they could take a deep breath of air this would relieve their distress. Many others are totally unaware of any changes in their breathing pattern. Being unaware of a change in breathing, they do not describe this to their doctor, and he may be unable to elicit the information even on questioning.

What happens in hyperventilation, whether people are aware that they are doing so or not, is that in more rapid breathing, the people blow off extra carbon dioxide. This may result in a significant change in the acid–base level of the blood.[1] The human body functions within a very narrow biochemical

[1]R. L. Rice, "Symptom Patterns of Hyperventilation Syndrome," *American Journal of Medicine* 8 (1950): 691–700; B. I. Lewis, "Hyperventilation Syndrome," *Annals Internal Medicine*, 38 (1953): 918–927; "Hyperventilation Syndrome," *Lancet* 2 (8313) (1982): 1438–1439.

range, and even minute changes in chemical balance can produce symptoms.

Exhaling excessive amounts of carbon dioxide makes the blood become more alkaline. This may create additional symptoms. The body may have slight change in some of the circulating minerals, and a change in the circulating calcium may occur. Frequent symptoms of these changes are twitching, irritability, numbness, and/or tingling of the fingers and the area around the lips, and occasionally spasms of the hands or feet. These symptoms may be very frightening, but when they are described to the physician, he can readily identify them as a sequelae of hyperventilation.

Sometimes these striking physical symptoms do not occur; instead the person exhibits primarily mental symptoms. Sometimes both types of symptoms occur together. The mental symptoms may be confusion, a feeling of unreality, a sense of depersonalization, giddiness, euphoria, or depression, or hallucinations.[2]

The phenomenon of hallucinating, either audially or visually, means that the person hears sounds that are nonexistent or sees things that are not there, respectively. Most people, mental health professionals included, generally associate hallucinating with psychosis, because hallucinations most frequently occur in schizophrenia. If the person shows no signs of ingesting alcohol or other drugs or any sign of brain disease or delerium, hallucinations are virtually always assumed to be symptoms of psychosis.

People who are sensitive to the changes in hyperventilation and who develop hallucinations may thus be misdiagnosed as psychotic. If they also have some mood changes with the hyperventilation, describe feelings of unreality, or experience the

[2]T. E. Allen and B. Agus, "Hyperventilation Leading to Hallucinations," *American Journal of Psychiatry* 125 (1968): 632–637; L. C. Lum, "Hyperventilation: The Tip of the Iceberg," *Journal of Psychosomatic Research* 19 (1975): 375-383.

sensation that their bodies are undergoing weird transformation, their being diagnosed as psychotic is very probable. If they are unaware that they are hyperventilating and do not arouse consideration of hyperventilation as a diagnosis by the physician, they may indeed be labeled and treated as psychotic, which may include hospitalization on a psychiatric unit and treatment with potent drugs. The latter experiences may themselves be traumatic if they are not absolutely necessary.

Various mental changes have been found to be brought on by hyperventilation, and although these cases may be very rare, the tragedy of misdiagnosis of psychosis is so great that this condition must be considered. Cases of multiple personality caused by hyperventilation have been described.[3]

A true psychosis does not last for a few minutes or an hour, then disappear and recur later. Brief episodes of unreality or hallucinating, with long intervals of normal mental functioning, should arouse the suspicion of hyperventilation. The symptoms may often be reproduced by voluntarily hyperventilating and may be relieved by breathing into a small paper bag, which allows people to rebreathe the exhaled carbon dioxide.

Treatment of recurrent anxiety attacks may not be simple, and the distress of these attacks may indeed be severe. However, there is no comparision between an anxiety neurosis and a psychosis. The latter can be a grave condition, and the diagnosis of a psychotic reaction may bring about major changes in the patient and his family, his occupation, and his entire life plan. With such gravity of consequences, the possibility that some very weird symptoms might be manifestations of hyperventilation needs to be considered.

---

[3]J. S. Silverman, "Multiple Personality as Sequel to Hyperventilation Syndrome," *American Journal of Psychiatry* 122 (1965): 217–220.

6

Thyroid
Disorders

The human body is an organism that is constantly active. Even during periods of rest, as in sleep, our bodies are churning with activity. The heart pumps blood, the lungs expand and contract, the digestive organs continue their functions, the kidney clears the blood of waste products, the liver manufactures the essential building blocks of tissue, the deepest portions of the brain regulate much of the activity, and, as is evident from the phenomenon of dreaming, even the thinking portions of the brain are at work. As long as the person is alive, every cell in the body is constantly biologically active.

There is, however, great variation in the rate at which the body functions. If one is very active physically and exercises strenuously, the body metabolism increases. The heart beats faster, breathing is more rapid, and chemical reactions accelerate to provide the body with the fuel for the increased activity. Similar changes occur in states of excitement or in febrile diseases. In all such instances, when the demand is over, the system returns to the slower rate of rest, referred to as the *basal metabolic rate.*

This may be understood by looking at the automobile engine. When one climbs a hill or travels at high speed, the engine must work harder; but when the car is in neutral, the motor runs at a slow rate. A little screw regulates this "idling rate." If this screw is turned up too high, the motor races even when the car is at rest, wasting gasoline and causing unnecessary wear of the engine parts. If the screw is turned too low, the motor sputters and stalls and may "die" at the most inopportune time, such as in the midst of a left turn in busy traffic.

The counterpart of the idling screw in the human body, which regulates the rate at which the body metabolizes at rest, is the thyroid gland. It produces the hormone *thyroxin*. If there is too much thyroxin in the circulation, the body is overactive even at rest; if there is too little thyroxin, a person does not have enough "get up and go," and the system "sputters and stalls."

Many of the symptoms of an overactive thyroid are those described in an anxiety attack. There is rapid heart rate with palpitation, sweating, tremor, insomnia, restlessness. If the thyroid is underactive, the person may feel sluggish, depressed, cold and clammy, without energy, and unable to concentrate. The symptoms of both anxiety and depression can thus be at times caused by improper thyroid function.

Obviously, if the cause of the problem is overactivity or underactivity of the thyroid, analyzing the patient's feelings and trying to treat the condition psychiatrically is going to be of little avail.

There are, of course, varying degrees of thyroid dysfunction. If the dysfunction is extreme, recognition should not be much of a problem. When the changes are less striking, the true condition may be overlooked. Once thyroid trouble is suspected, the correct diagnosis can be made by a simple blood test.

Sometimes even an extreme case can escape the notice of a physician. If the patient has thyroid deficiency, and the physician is not struck by the patient's appearance on their first encounter, it is possible that he may not think of the diagnosis on subsequent visits because he thinks that this is the patient's normal appearance.

Stella was fifty-two and a widow six years. Her husband had died of a heart attack, and she sustained herself with a small pension that complemented her Social Security benefits. Her house was totally paid for. Stella had one daughter, who was married to a career Navy officer, and they lived some two thousand miles away.

Stella had made a satisfactory adjustment to her situation. She worked as an "extra" sales clerk at a department store and was called on in busy seasons or to replace an absentee. She worked at the polling places at election time. She attended church regularly and assisted with "Meals on Wheels."

For several months, Stella had felt somewhat "down." She did not have the same "zip." She had turned down calls to help with "Meals on Wheels" and on one occasion even rejected a work opportunity at the store. However, she did not think anything was wrong with her and saw no reason to consult her physician.

One day, Stella slipped while getting out of the bathtub and struck her ribs. The pain was intense, and she called her doctor. X-rays revealed two broken ribs, and the doctor prescribed a binder and some pain medication.

When the doctor asked her how she had been doing otherwise, Stella confided that she had not been feeling up to par. The doctor asked whether she had hot flashes, which she had indeed experienced, and he then told her that she was having fairly typical menopausal symptoms, which could be relieved by hormone medication. These were prescribed, and she was to return to the doctor in three months.

Stella took the medication as prescribed and found that the hot flashes did indeed subside. However, her other symptoms became more intense. She became listless and much more depressed. Everything that had previously interested her no longer held her attention. She spent many hours in bed, getting up only to do the bare minimum in the house.

When Stella returned for her three-month followup, she told the doctor how she was feeling. The doctor said that she was having a menopausal depression and arranged for an appointment with a psychiatrist.

The psychiatrist recorded Stella's symptoms and took a fairly extensive history. He confirmed the doctor's diagnostic impression of menopausal depression and prescribed an anti-depressant medication. He also told Stella that she was suffering from the "empty–nest syndrome," with her husband gone and her one daughter living so far away. Stella asked why this had not affected her previously, because she had been alone for six years, and the psychiatrist explained that the combination of physical and situational factors produced the depression. He assured Stella that the medication would relieve her depression within a few weeks and suggested that she go in to see him once weekly.

Stella felt that the sessions with the psychiatrist were beneficial and that she did have an opportunity to talk about her loneliness. When three weeks passed with no change in the way she felt, the psychiatrist prescribed a different antidepressant medication. Her depression remained unaffected by the second antidepressant, and at the psychiatrist's recommendation, Stella entered a hospital for electroshock treatments.

Stella did not remember much about the hospitalization. She returned home after a four-week hospitalization during which she had received six treatments. She continued to see the psychiatrist weekly, but instead of improving, her condition deteriorated. The psychiatrist then advised rehospitalization, and a few days after admission, he told Stella that she would require long-term treatment and that the state hospital was the only place this was available.

The mention of the state hospital was very upsetting to Stella. She had visions of entering and never leaving, being under the impression that this was the place where people were "put away." The psychiatrist assured her that this would not be so in her case but that she might require several months of hospitalization. Stella realized that she had little choice. The way she was feeling, she could not manage on her own.

After being admitted to the state hospital, Stella was told

by her new doctor that he was going to prescribe a different medication that he believed would be effective. Stella was also to participate in occupational therapy and industrial therapy. She was assigned a job in the hospital cannery.

Stella often refused to report for her assigned job, and initially this was overlooked because the doctor thought the medication had not yet had a chance to work. When nothing changed after several weeks of the new medication, Stella's doctor told her that she should have a course of electroshock treatment. Stella explained that a previous course of treatments had not helped, and the doctor said that this was because six treatments were not sufficient. He felt that perhaps twelve treatments would be necessary to relieve her depression.

After another three months the course of treatments was completed, and still Stella felt no different. She was then transferred from the acute treatment unit to the chronic building.

My personal contact with Stella occurred about two years after this. I had joined the staff of the state hospital and had been assigned to a chronic unit that housed approximately 300 patients. To familiarize myself with the patients who would be under my care, I arranged to review the records of ten patients each day and, following the review of each record, arranged to meet with each patient for a brief personal contact.

When Stella came in for her interview, my immediate reaction was, "My God, she's myxedematous."[1] The expression of her face, the dry skin, the sparse, brittle hair, and the hoarse voice all pointed to severe thyroid deficiency. A quick testing of her reflexes further supported this diagnosis, which was subsequently confirmed by laboratory studies.

Review of earlier medical records indicated a moderate anemia, and I had every reason to suspect that the thyroid deficiency had existed all the way back. Thyroid function studies had not been done in any previous hospitalization.

[1]Myxedema is a condition resulting from low thyroid function.

Thyroid replacement was instituted in very small doses and increased very gradually, because a rapid increase in metabolism would have overtaxed her heart. After three months, the changes in Stella were dramatic. Instead of sitting aimlessly on a bench or walking the long corridors of the hospital all day, Stella became an early riser. She was transferred to the convalescent unit and took a job in the "Little Store" that was part of the hospital complex.

Stella did not make the move from the hospital back to the community. Two years of state hospital confinement had made her totally reliant on the hospital. There was no one in the community to give her the kind of support she would have needed to reestablish an independent existence. When I left the service of the state hospital two years later, Stella had decided to stay on indefinitely.

Lesser degrees of over- or under-activity of the thyroid may not be evident by the patient's appearance or even on physical examination. Careful questioning can elicit information that can direct the physician to the correct diagnosis. If the patient is not adequately evaluated, these conditions can easily be missed.[2]

The relationship of thyroid to emotion is a two-way affair. As noted, thyroid dysfunction can bring about significant emotional symptoms. However, emotional changes may actually precipitate a thyroid disorder. It has been observed that overactivity of the thyroid is often preceded by an emotional upset.

Patients who have a *bona fide emotional* disorder and who are treated appropriately for it may thus subsequently develop thyroid dysfunction in the course of therapy. Unless the therapist remains alert to this possibility, the patient's poor progress in treatment may be erroneously attributed to psychological factors. Because prolonged overactivity or underactivity of the thyroid

[2]M. S. Gold and H. R. Pearsall, "Hypothyroidism, or Is It Depression?" *Psychosomatics* 24 (7) (July 1983): 646–655.

may also bring about serious physical damage, the need for acute alertness during the course of psychiatric treatment is evident.

Whereas the symptoms of overactive thyroid are quite classic and present little diagnostic challenge, at times nature pulls one of its "atypical" tricks, and the patient does not present the symptoms that the student was taught in medical school. Because "atypical" cases are infrequent, they are more likely to be misdiagnosed.

Nancy was fifty-eight, married and the mother of three children, all of whom were grown and married. Her husband was sixty-three and had just recently retired from the steel mill. Nancy had gone through a rather uneventful menopause several years earlier. She now began to feel somewhat depressed, began losing interest in things, and lost her appetite.

Ed and Nancy had looked forward to his retirement as a time when they would be able to do some of the things they had dreamt of earlier. Especially, they were going to tour the country coast-to-coast in their trailer. Nancy's depression and lethargy put a damper on their plans, much to the disappointment of both.

Nancy consulted a psychiatrist, who prescribed antidepressant medication. She showed little if any improvement, and several courses of different antidepressants were tried without result. Nancy lost weight and became progressively weaker. The psychiatrist then referred her to an internist, who hospitalized her for evaluation.

Because of the weakness and lethargy, the internist felt that Nancy might be thyroid deficient, and although she did not manifest the usual physical signs of an underactive thyroid, he ordered thyroid function tests. He was surprised, therefore, to find that the tests indicated that Nancy had an *overactive* thyroid. Further tests confirmed the diagnosis of thyrotoxicosis.

Nancy was treated with radioactive iodine, and over a period of several months her depression improved, her appetite returned, and she regained the lost weight.

7

Caffeinism

As an inveterate coffee lover, I am distressed to have to implicate this wonderful beverage as a cause of symptoms of emotional illness. Yet what is now a scientifically established fact must be recognized: coffee sometimes *can* cause trouble. We are apt to take this quite lightly and perhaps joke about it while sipping a cup, but to the person who is incapacitated by frequent anxiety attacks or who is not responding to treatment for a severe agitated depression, this is deadly serious business.

The culprit in coffee is, of course, its caffeine. Caffeine is also present in significant quantities in tea, in colas, and in over-the-counter medications and stimulants.

People react in a great variety of ways to different psychoactive drugs. For example, not everyone who uses alcohol becomes dependent on it or suffers harmful effects. Similarly, many people may be able to consume caffeine-containing drinks without ill effects, particularly if they use caffeine in moderation. Some people however, may be sensitive to relatively small amounts of caffeine. Very sensitive people may have negative effects from coffee with as little as two cups in the morning. On the other hand, many people consume far too much caffeine.

Caffeine is a rather powerful stimulant. It affects all parts of the brain, thus not only affecting the state of alertness, but also the circulation and respiration. Caffeine may increase the heart rate and the force of the heart contraction. It increases the output and strength of acid in the stomach, and, as demonstrated by the increased frequency of urination, it affects the kidneys. A chemical with such widespread effects on the body cannot be dismissed lightly.[1]

The stimulant effects of caffeine may result in headaches, hyperventilation, twitching, and feelings of jitters and restlessness. Rapid heart rate, episodes of palpitation, and irregular heart rhythm may occur. Insomnia is a common effect.[2] People who are depressed and who feel sluggish may take caffeine-containing products to give them a lift.[3] This may convert the depression from a sluggish depression to an agitated depression, wherein the person still feels very dejected but now finds himself restless and unable to sit still for very long.

Understandably, people who feel jittery and nervous may try to get relief with tranquilizers. However, the caffeine may counteract the action of the tranquilizer, and the dosage of tranquilizer may be increased, thus leading to the possibility of addiction.

A cup of brewed coffee contains between 100 mg and 150 mg of caffeine, and instant coffee has slightly less, 85 mg to 100 mg per cup. Tea is about 60 mg to 75 mg per cup, and a glass of cola has about 40 mg to 60 mg. Prescribed medication for headache and other pain, as well as over-the-counter medications, may have between 40 mg and 60 mg per tablet, and the "keep-awake" type of pills contain approximately 100 mg per tablet. Decaffeinated coffee has only 2 mg to 4 mg per cup.

Phyllis is a twenty-seven-year-old nurse who was married to an army physician. She had adjusted well to military life but

[1]B. S. Victor, M. Lubitsky, and J. F. Greden, "Somatic Manifestation of Caffeinism," *Journal of Clinical Psychiatry* 42 (1981): 185–188.

[2]J. M. Ritchie, *Central Nervous Systems Stimulants, II: The Xanthines*, in the *Pharmacological Basis of Therapeutics*, 4th ed. Edited by L. S. Goodman and A. Gilman, (New York: MacMillan Publishing Co., 1970), 358-370; R. Erhardt, "Psychic Disturbances in Caffeine Intoxication," *Acta Med. Scand.*, 71 (1929): 94–99.

[3]J. F. Neil, "Caffeinism Complicating Hypersomnic Depressive Episodes," *Comprehensive Psychiatry*, Vol. 19, (1978): 377–385.

had recently become concerned that her husband might be transferred to Vietnam.

Throughout the stresses of nursing school and on her job, Phyllis had always taken things in stride. She considered herself quite capable of handling stress situations, and in the hospital she was known as someone who "kept her cool" even when pressures were intense. She was therefore surprised when she began to develop symptoms that she recognized as anxiety.

Phyllis had begun to experience headaches and sensations of lightheadedness. She had initially dismissed these as probably caused by a virus, although she did not have any of the usual cold symptoms. She then noticed that occasionally her hands would shake with a very fine tremor. A few days later, she felt like something was "jumping" inside her chest. She applied her stethoscope to her chest and was alarmed to discover that her heartbeat was irregular. After perhaps ten beats or so, two "extra" beats would occur. Phyllis had never experienced any heart irregularity previously and consulted a physician.

The doctor found no abnormality on examination or in her blood tests. The electrocardiograph, however, did confirm that she had an irregular heart rhythm.

The doctor questioned Phyllis about possible upsetting events in her life. Phyllis admitted that she had some understandable apprehension about her husband possibly being transferred to Vietnam, but she did not feel that she was reacting with anxiety symptoms because she had never before "fallen apart" under stress. The doctor said that the possibility of being separated from her husband, especially if he were sent to a combat zone, was qualitatively different than any other stress she had experienced heretofore. He recommended that Phyllis discuss her problem with a psychiatrist.

Phyllis returned home, unconvinced of the doctor's diagnosis. She thought of her father's death when she was about fifteen and of how she had been supportive to her mother through the ordeal. She remembered how she had reacted with efficiency and stability the second week she was on duty in the hospital when a cardiac arrest occurred and how her superiors had commended her for taking things in control.

Phyllis sat in her kitchen, trying to figure out what had happened during the past three weeks that was different. As she went to pour herself a cup of coffee, she stopped abruptly. It was just a little over three weeks that John had bought her a new coffee-maker for Valentine's Day. Before that she had used instant coffee and had drunk perhaps three or four cups daily. But this new coffee was so much better and the aroma of brewed coffee was so enticing that she had increased her coffee drinking to about ten cups a day. Could it be that this change in her diet was responsible for her symptoms?

There was only one way to find out, Phyllis thought. She would eliminate coffee completely and see what happened.

The first day of abstinence was uneventful, but on the second day Phyllis felt as though she weighed a ton. She had difficulty getting out of bed and getting things done. She applied the stethoscope to her chest: No "extra" beats, just a regular rhythm.

On the following day, Phyllis felt much better. No fatigue, no headache, no heart flutter. She then asked the doctor to repeat the electrocardiograph: Rhythm regular, no extra beats. She told the doctor about her diagnosis, but the doctor was unconvinced, and again recommended that she see a psychiatrist.

After ten days with no recurrence of anxiety symptoms, Phyllis decided that her diagnosis had to be confirmed. She brewed a fresh pot of coffee and drank eight cups. She continued this for several days, and on the third day she felt the familiar heart flutter. She applied the stethoscope, and she again had the extra beats. She went to the doctor and had another cardiogram taken that demonstrated the irregular rhythm. This time the doctor was convinced.

Phyllis gave the coffee-maker an early retirement from active duty and has had no recurrence of any symptoms.

As noted, some sensitive people may be affected by as little as 250 mg per day of caffeine.[4] A person who has four cups of brewed coffee during the day, takes two tablets of a common, over-the-counter headache pill twice a day, and has a can of cola may thus be ingesting more than 800 mg caffeine in a twenty-four-hour period. Certainly people who drink more than eight cups of regular coffee per day are consuming enough caffeine to cause symptoms. In retrospect, I think about a young man who was hospitalized, diagnosed, and treated for schizophrenia. Even while in the hospital, he used to drink at least fifteen cans of cola daily in addition to coffee. He thus ingested at least 1,200 mg caffeine daily, and I can only wonder whether he was indeed schizophrenic or rather psychotoxic with caffeine. At least one case of caffeine psychosis has been reported.[5]

Stopping the consumption of coffee or other caffeine-containing substances may appear to be a simple if unwelcome solution. Unfortunately, things are a bit more complicated. People who are accustomed to caffeine may experience some very distressing symptoms when they stop using it. These are genuine withdrawal symptoms, and these may consist of severe headache, irritability, inability to work effectively, and restlessness.[6]

A comic strip used to advertise a coffee-substitute beverage that featured a malicious-looking villain called "Mr. Coffee Nerves," who used to shoot poison arrows at someone about to engage in some pleasurable activity. Whereas many people

[4]W. Silver, "Insomnia, Tachycardia and Cola Drinks," *Pediatrics* 47 (1971): 635–637.

[5]E. G. Truitt, "The Xanthines," in *Drills Pharmacology in Medicine*, 4th Ed. Edited by Dipalma, (New York: Macmillan Publishing Co., 1970), 358–370; M. C. McManamy and P. G. Shube, "Caffeine Intoxication: Report of a Case the Symptoms of Which Amounted to a Psychosis," *New England Journal of Medicine*, 215 (1936): 616–620.

[6]A. Goldstein and S. Kaizer, "Psychotropic Effects of Caffeine in Man, III: A Questionnaire Survey of Coffee Drinkers and Its Effects in a Group of Housewives," *Clinical Pharmacology Therapy*, 10 (1969): 477–488; R. H. Driesbach and C. Pfeiffer, "Caffeine-Withdrawal Headache," *Journal of Laboratory Clinical Medicine*, 28 (1943): 1212–1218.

probably can use coffee in moderation without ill effects, people who do have symptoms that could result from caffeine ingestion must consider this possibility, certainly before concluding that they have a mental condition that requires treatment. People may have to stop using caffeine-containing products gradually to avoid the distressing withdrawal symptoms; then they must allow a period of at least several weeks without caffeine to elapse to evaluate the possible cause–effect relationship.

Because anxiety can be self-reinforcing, the overall effect of caffeine-induced anxiety may be much greater than its pure chemical effects.[7]

[7]Y. Gilliland and D. Andress, "Ad Lib Caffeine Consumption, Symptoms of Caffeinism, and Academic Performance," *American Journal of Psychiatry,* 138 (1981): 512–514; J. A. Sours, "Case Report of Anorexia Nervosa and Caffeinism," *American Journal of Psychiatry,* 140 (1983): 235–236.

8

Hypoglycemia, Diabetes, and Nutrition

The role of hypoglycemia, or low blood sugar, as a cause of psychological symptoms is controversial. Some writers for the lay public have attributed many symptoms to low blood sugar and consider it one of the most overlooked disorders. They claim that lack of proper diagnosis of hypoglycemia has frequently resulted in labeling the patient as "neurotic" and in unnecessary and ineffective treatment.[1] On the other hand, articles in the medical literature tend to minimize hypoglycemia as a frequent cause of symptoms, unless the blood sugar levels are dangerously low.[2] As in many other instances with two extremes, the truth probably lies somewhere in the middle.[3]

It is universally agreed that when the blood sugar level is extremely low, various symptoms characteristic of mental illness can occur. This is most likely to happen to diabetics who take insulin or other medications to lower their blood sugar level

[1]E. Fredericks and H. Goodman, *Low Blood Sugar and You*. (New York: Charter Books, 1969); W. A. Nolen, "Low Blood Sugar—What It Means," MaCalls, 103; G. B. Kolata, "The Truth About Hypoglycemia," MS, 8:26. E. M. Abrahamson and A. W. Pexet, *Body, Mind, and Sugar*, (New York: Pyramid Communications, 1951).

[2]J. Leggett and A. R. Favazza, "Hypoglycemia, An Overview," *Journal of Clinical Psychiatry*, (January 1978) 51–57; D. D. Johnson, K. E. Door, W. M. Swenson, and J. Service, "*Reactive Hypoglycemia*," *Journal of American Medical Association*, 243 (1980): 1151.

[3]F. Hale, S. Margen, and D. Rabak, "Postprandial Hypoglycemia and Psychological Symptoms," "*Biological Psychiatry* 17 (1981): 125–129.

and who are either unstable, forget to eat, or have excessive physical exertion. Generally diabetics and their families are alerted to these possibilities, but exceptions can occur.

The hospital with which I am affiliated has for years been providing medical and surgical services for a state hospital whose patients may require more intensive physical treatment. Usually, the patient would be admitted to the medical or surgical service. But, on occasion, the state hospital would ask that the patient be housed on the psychiatric unit for security reasons while he was undergoing the indicated medical care.

One time I received a call from the state hospital about a man of thirty-seven who had fractured his forearm while beating his hands against the wall in a rage outburst. I was asked to keep him on the psychiatric unit while he underwent the surgical treatment, because he was "too aggressive and uncontrollable" for the general hospital.

Several days after the patient had undergone the necessary orthopedic procedure, the nurse on the psychiatric unit told me that it was strange that this man was in a state mental hospital, because he appeared to be so normal. After interviewing the patient, I had to agree with the nurse, and on reviewing the medical record, I found that the patient was a diabetic who was receiving insulin. I then delayed the patient's return to the state hospital and left orders that in the event the patient showed any signs of abnormal behavior whatsoever, a prompt blood-sugar level was to be determined.

During the next few days, he had two episodes of severe agitation. Blood samples drawn during those instances showed extremely low blood-sugar levels.

I then called the patient's wife for additional information, and she told me that she had been instructed to give the patient orange juice if he began to behave strangely. One time, however, he had become very enraged and combative and had refused to take the orange juice. He then became so disturbed that she had to call a police ambulance. When he was examined in a hospital emergency room, he was immediately diagnosed as "crazy" and was promptly transferred to the state hospital, where he had remained for two months until the incident occurred where he broke his forearm.

Needless to say, this patient was not returned to the state hospital. His insulin dosage was regulated, and he was discharged to his family.

It is frightening to consider that if not for the fracture, this young man might have spent many years in a mental institution, although he was in no way mentally ill.

The majority of cases of low blood sugar are not of this kind but are referred to as "reactive" or "functional" hypoglycemia. For reasons that are not too clear, some people's sugar metabolism is not precise—it appears that their bodies' output of insulin overshoots the mark, resulting in a lowering of the blood sugar. This may give rise to symptoms of nausea, profuse sweating, tremors, dizziness, and confusion. The drop in blood sugar may also trigger a release of adrenalin, with the resultant symptoms of an anxiety attack as described earlier. This is apt to occur in people who have a family history of diabetes.

People with low blood sugar symptoms often empirically discover that eating a candy bar or other sweets will temporarily relieve their symptoms. The problem is that this relief is often shortlived, because the body is apt to handle this newly ingested sugar with an outpouring of too much insulin, resulting in another attack.

On the other hand, the anxiety episode may come first and may bring in its wake a hypoglycemic episode. It is often difficult to distinguish which is the chicken and which is the egg. Whichever comes first, a self-perpetuating cycle can occur.

Even in those instances where the anxiety precedes the hypoglycemia, the initial emotional reaction might have been self-limited or much more easily managed if the vicious cycle were not set in motion. The ultimate panic reaction may be grossly out of proportion to the original stimulus. People may seek relief of the intense symptoms by tranquilizing themselves with alcohol, which unfortunately often aggravates the hypoglycemia. They may consult their physician or a psychiatrist, and unless the role of hypoglycemia is recognized and the proper dietary correction instituted, the people may be overmedicated with possibly addicting tranquilizers, or overtreated psychotherapeutically. They may indeed be misdiagnosed as neurotic.

The diagnosis of hypoglycemia should be carefully considered, because an error in either direction can be harmful. Wrongly attributing everything to hypoglycemia is just as unwise as overlooking hypoglycemia. Certainly a six-hour glucose tolerance test is worthwhile, and there is no harm in a few weeks' trial on a low-carbohydrate–high-protein diet to see if this relieves any of the patient's symptoms.

One might think that diabetes would not be mistaken as mental illness, because it is relatively simple to diagnose, but there is room for error. Diabetes does not always present the classical symptoms of thirst, weight loss, and frequent urination. The only symptoms of diabetes may be fatigue or sexual impotence, and obviously these can be mistaken as symptoms of depression. Even a single negative blood or urine test does not necessarily rule out diabetes. A careful history and physical examination followed by the necessary laboratory studies will clarify the diagnosis.

Edwin was a thirty-eight-year-old man who was admitted to the hospital because of alcohol intoxication. After the acute symptoms receded, he gave the following history.

Edwin said that he had never drunk excessively until the past year. Prior to that, he drank infrequently and even then only minimal amounts of alcohol. Two years earlier, he had begun to have difficulties with sexual impotence.

About three years before the sexual problem began, Edwin and his wife underwent a serious marital crisis when she admitted to him that she had been having an extramarital relationship. For a while, it appeared that they were going to divorce.

However, they sought marital counseling, and the marriage was maintained. Sexual relations returned to normal until the impotence began.

When the impotence occurred, Edwin returned to the marriage counselor for help and was advised that impotence is not an unusual occurrence following a trying period in the marriage. The counselor did not feel any therapy was necessary at that time. He told Edwin that although he had forgiven his wife, he was still harboring some deep resentments, which were responsible for his impotence. He said that these resentments and the sexual difficulty would disappear.

As the sexual problem persisted, Edwin began to be more critical of his wife, holding her indiscretions responsible for his problem. Repeated discussions became progressively more belligerent, until the couple finally reached a tacit agreement to drop the subject. By this time, their communication had deteriorated, and they became distant from each other.

Edwin said that about this time, he began stopping at a bar after work. He was not looking forward to a cold and even hostile environment at home. The bar provided him with companionship and with a chemical that tranquilized his frayed nerves. As time progressed, his drinking increased.

The routine blood tests performed when Edwin was admitted to the hospital showed a marked elevation of the blood sugar. Since this can occur as an aftermath of heavy drinking, the test was repeated after four days of abstinence and was again abnormal. Doctors then learned that Edwin's grandmother and two uncles had been diabetic. His father had died of a heart attack at age forty-two, and although no one knew whether he had been diabetic, there were grounds for assuming this. Edwin was told to totally abstain from alcohol and to consult a physician for further evaluation.

Edwin abstained from alcohol, and subsequent evaluation established that he was indeed diabetic. With appropriate management of the diabetes, Edwin had moderate improvement of his sexual performance, albeit not a complete return to normal.

There was every reason to believe that the major factor in Edwin's impotence was the diabetes rather than the emotional component. Indeed, the impotence resulting from the diabetes became the contributing factor for the deterioration of the marriage after the reconciliation and for the depression and frustration that led to Edwin's turning toward alcohol.

Whereas true vitamin deficiencies are not frequent, even in this day and age of enriched foods people can have vitamin deficiencies. Even people who are obese can be vitamin deficient. People who have special diets, such as for peptic ulcer, or people who have certain food eccentricities may be deficient in one or more vitamins. People who use alcohol to excess (a highly relative term) may have very real deficiencies of some of the B vitamins. Such deficiencies may cause irritability, depression, fatigue, and anxiety—all easily mistaken for emotional disorders. No psychotherapy, tranquilizer, or antidepressant can be effective as long as these deficiencies persist.

The role of nutrition in emotional symptomatology is unclear. Nutrition has undoubtedly been commercially exploited, and many people are probably spending money on expensive health foods and/or swallowing vitamins, minerals, and dietary supplements that they do not need. On the other hand, I doubt whether most physicians are well-versed in nutrition. All I can say is that unless other physicians have learned a great deal more about nutrition than I was taught in my medical school education, they know pitiably little.

Food faddists will have us believe that we are what we eat. While this is an overstatement, nutrition cannot be lightly dismissed, and there is no reason to believe that what we consume every day has no impact on our physical or mental functioning. One does not have to be an expert on nutrition to conclude that the current dietary practices of our culture, replete with junk foods and fast foods, probably do not provide optimally for our bodies' needs. The cultural obsession with providing as much gratification of our senses as we possibly can has undoubtedly resulted in some unhealthy eating habits. Yet, except when certain diseases require specific diets, many physicians do not take a detailed nutritional history nor would they know what to do about modifying the patient's nutritional regimen.

The lack of adequate teaching about nutrition in medical schools is just one aspect of a prevailing philosophy in medical education. Except for instruction in immunization, relatively little attention is given to prevention and to preservation of health, as contrasted to treatment of illnesses. The consequences of this is that many physicians know a great deal about diseases but relatively little about health.

This attitude has had an obvious consequence in psychiatry. The psychiatrist must complete the standard medical curriculum before going on to specialized training in psychological problems. Like his other medical colleagues who look for the infecting bacteria or virus, the disturbed metabolism, or the malignant cell, he, too, is oriented to look for pathology, and he does so when patients present themselves to him with emotional symptoms. As if by reflex, the psychiatrist in his evaluation and history-taking of the patient looks for the childhood deprivations and other emotional traumata that may have contributed to the patient's problems.

Whereas this type of thinking certainly has its place, many patients consult a psychiatrist because of faulty adapations they are making to their life's situations because they lack the awareness that they have the skills, strengths, and capacity to cope effectively. What they need to improve their functioning is not a discovery of what went wrong with them in their development but rather an awareness of their personality resources and a strengthening of their coping skills. In other words, rather than being helped to find out what is *wrong* with them, they should be helped to discover what is *right* with them. Just as people with weak, flabby muscles can improve their strength by appropriate exercises that enable them to maximize their potential that already exists within their muscles, so the people with inadequate coping skills need to learn how to maximize the potential that is within them in terms of their intellectual and personality resources. Unfortunately, a pathology–oriented psychiatric physician may gravitate to focusing on the areas of emotional pathology rather than also directing his attention toward improving the patient's underdeveloped skills.[1]

Psychotherapy, both individual and group, can be directed toward greater self-awareness and improvement of one's coping skills. Self-help groups are often available that help people strengthen their inherent potentials. These should be used to the fullest when the patients' needs are amenable to that kind of group support, and the groups can complement formal psychotherapy as well as eliminate pathological conflicts.

[4]In my book *Like Yourself, . . . and Others Will Too* (Prentice-Hall, 1978), I described numerous examples of psychological problems resulting from the individual's underevaluation of himself.

Alcohol and Drugs

The terms "normal" and "average" are sometimes interchanged as though they were synonymous. Yet this is clearly not so. If a population were infected with tuberculosis and most of its people died before fifty, the "average" life span might be forty-four or so, and it might be "average" to harbor active tuberculosis, but this would in no way be "normal." The fact that a condition is extremely prevalent may indeed make it fairly average, but prevalence says nothing about normality.

The use of mood-altering chemicals in our culture is extremely widespread, and although alcohol heads the list, many other chemicals, both prescribed and over-the-counter are widely consumed.

The chemicals I am referring to, alcohol included, are consumed for one reason and for one reason only: they bring about a change of feeling. The change may be the "glow" of alcohol, relaxing or sedative effect, its relieving a state of tension, or its making one more convivial. The change may be the sedative or tension-relieving effect of the tranquilizers or sleeping pill, or the stimulating or exhiliarating effect of the diet pill or marijuana.

Obviously, mood-altering drugs can be effective in only one way—by affecting brain function and doing something to cells of the brain. Any drug that does not alter brain function will not provide the sought-after effect.

In spite of our colloquialisms that emotions originate in

the heart, (I love you with my *heart*; my *heart* aches for him; please accept my *heart*felt gratitude) all emotions reside in the brain, as do also our reasoning, intellect, judgment, and memory. Any chemical that can affect the brain can affect all these brain-dependent functions.

The effects of excessive amounts of alcohol are well--known, but the prevalence of excessive drinking is still grossly under-estimated. The figures that are generally given for the incidence of alcoholism refer to drinkers who have begun to manifest symptoms of alcohol excess, whether they be physical deteriora-tion, gross mental aberration, social and domestic maladjust-ments, or trouble on the job. At least an equal number of excessive drinkers experience negative effects of alcohol that have not been sufficiently dramatic or disruptive to warrant classification under the current definition of alcoholism.

Not enough people recognize that many people may not qualify as alcoholic under the prevailing definition, but their emotional status is definitely impaired by alcohol. They may be consuming what is considered a "moderate" amount of alcohol, and their drinking may be "average." Please remember that "average" does does not mean "normal."

Although drunken driving laws consider drivers guilty only if they have a certain concentration of alcohol in their blood (usually a minimum of 0.1 percent), some people are affected by lesser amounts, with more subtle but definite changes in coordination and in reflex–response time. Because driving may be impaired by even fraction-of-a-second delays in reflex response and by minor impediments in judgment and co-ordination, unsafe driving may result when the blood alcohol level is below the legally established limit.

Similarly, subtle changes in emotional functioning may be caused by quantities of alcohol that do not result in gross drunkenness. Inhibitions may be loosened, with erotic or aggres-sive behavior emerging. People may become more irritable or belligerent and argumentative toward significant people in their environment, such as family members or employers. Their judgment may be impaired, with them making unwise decisions that they might have avoided with greater clarity of thought. Although such reactions occur under the influence of alcohol, in the absence of gross drunkenness, they may not be attributed to alcohol, and the erotic, aggressive, or belligerent behavior may be taken as representing people's true attitudes.

I would like to digress a bit at this point to say a few words about repression.

Philosophically, I consider humans to be unique beings, composed of essentially animal bodies, but endowed with a spirit that makes them capable of achieving a degree of mastery over the animalistic drives. Thus, whereas an animal's behavior is determined by its impulses and its strengths, countered by external obstacles to the gratification of its cravings, humans have an additional element: a spirit or conscience or code of living, which enables mature humans to have internal control over their behavior.

According to this concept, humans have many protoplasmic urges that may be lustful, acquisitive, or hostile. Without the controls that develop as they mature, humans would essentially be animals, capable of doing whatever animals do. Some behavioral controls are exerted consciously: for example, people are aware of urges to do particular actions and knowingly and volitionally restrain themselves. Other controls are deeply ingrained, especially those learned early in life, and become automatic behavioral restraints. In the latter instances, people may not even be aware that they are restraining themselves from carrying out particular impulses.

Both the voluntary and automatic controls are learned behavior and thus are superimposed upon a group of biological drives that are inherent in people. Chemicals that depress brain activity always depress learned behavior (the "higher functions") before they affect biological drives. Thus alcohol, which is a brain-tissue depressant, first depresses people's systems of controls, permitting uninhibited emergence of underlying drives.

The above description is an oversimplification of the human control system and its response to alcohol. Numerous other factors, such as varying intensities of repression of different drives, or effects of other associated emotions, enter into a complex system that ultimately determines which behavior emerges and in what form it emerges.

Generally, alcohol does not "create" behavior but rather uninhibits people so that underlying drives can emerge. Yet, it would be naive and incorrect to say that behaviors that emerge under the influence of alcohol are people's "true personalities," unless "true personality" means the naked human biological drives, in which case all our "true personalities" are similar. People's "true personalities" are the sum total of their innate drives *plus* all the maturation that they undergo as a result of learning, training, and experience. All we can say about alcohol-induced behavior is that it is a manifestation of many forces that are operative within individuals, some of which are now under lesser restraint. While some people who are normally polite and pleasant may became aggressive and obnoxious under the influence of alcohol, people whose usual attitude is belligerent and irritating may also become pleasant and friendly after drinking.

The popular view of the effects of alcohol is often more simplistic. People are apt to discount what a person says or does when he is clearly intoxicated, such as, "that's not really him, that's the booze talking out of him. In real life, you can't find a better person." Furthermore, the drinker himself, although he may be full of remorse over his drunken behavior, is also likely to dismiss this as something alien to him.

However, when people consume alcohol but are *not* clearly intoxicated, they are held much more accountable for their behaviors, which are considered as reflecting their "real selves." Similarly, "moderate" drinkers who do not have amnesia for their behavior and consider themselves to have been under perfect control, do not dismiss their behavior as being alien to their true personalities.

All this results in a kind of paradox, because "moderate" drinking may thus cause even greater difficulties than severe inebriation. An insult or offense occurring under gross inebriation is more apt to be forgiven, and the drinker is more likely to apologize. "I'm sorry about what happened the other night, Bill. Cheez, I don't even remember saying that. I was shocked when Ellen told me about it the next day. You know that wasn't me talking."

On the other hand, when drinkers are not obviously drunk, both they and those about them are not apt to dismiss their behavior so lightly. Furthermore, drinkers recall what they said and the circumstances under which they said it, and rather than apologize, they may be more likely to rationalize and try to justify their actions. An offensive remark can thus become a nidus for disruption of communication and deterioration of a relationship. Drinking is often the beginning of the ruination of a marriage. With the heavy drinker, the spouse is apt to recognize the problem as alcohol-related, but the "moderate" drinker's behavior is generally considered to be his "true self."

Alcohol and drugs can also produce depressive feelings, and withdrawal from these substances can bring about classic anxiety symptoms, with tremors, palpitations, and insomnia. Again, in contrast to the one-fifth per day or half-case-beer per day drinkers, people who have been drinking "moderately" and those close to them are unlikely to attribute the emotional changes to alcohol withdrawal and may believe that they have some other type of mental illness.

No guidelines to "safe" quantities can be given. People's vulnerability to the effects of alcohol and drugs differ greatly. Some people are very sensitive to relatively small amounts of mood-altering substances, and there is no way to sort them out.

People who undergo emotional changes secondary to "moderate" use of alcohol or drugs, or the couple whose marriage is deteriorating and who seek professional help with their problems, may get into further difficulty if the role of the mood-altering chemical is not discovered. If the daily drinking is in "moderation," patients are most unlikely to volunteer any information about their alcohol use. Too often, therapists do not inquire carefully about the use of alcohol or other drugs, and even if they do, they are apt to accept an answer such as "I have a social drink" at its face value. Patients who have two martinis at lunch, one or two at dinner, and three to four ounces during the evening may indeed believe their drinking to be "social" and innocuous, and therapists are often apt to concur. The therapy then begins to focus on other goings-on in the patients' lives, and multiple areas of dissatisfaction begin to be investigated. Some of these may be given undue significance, and, particularly in marriages, areas of "conflict" may be magnified out of proportion. Alcohol and drugs, either in gross excess or in "moderation" are without a doubt more responsible for family dissolution than any other single factor and possibly even more than all other factors combined.

If the role of alcohol and/or drugs as causes of or contributors to patients' problems is not recognized, and patients are believed to have a depressive or psychoneurotic condition, physicians may prescribe antidepressants and/or tranquilizers. While these medications can be very effective in appropriate cases, their effects in cases that are complicated by alcohol or drugs can range from worthless to disastrous. Alcohol or drugs may prevent the prescribed medication from having its therapeutic effects, and if patients continue to use alcohol together with the prescribed medication, the interaction between the two can be dangerous. I have seen innumerable cases where psychiatric treatment was continued for years with complete futility because therapists were unaware of the patients' drinking or did not consider it to be of any significance.

Some drugs may produce mental symptoms that are indistinguishable from serious mental illnesses. Amphetamines, often used, or better yet, *mis*used for diet control or for staying awake, may produce hallucinations and delusions that may closely mimic schizophrenia. Discontinuance of these drugs may result in severe depressions. Both of these conditions are generally self-limited and respond well to treatment, but many complications can result if they are misdiagnosed as schizophrenia or psychotic depression rather than as a reaction to a drug.

Cathy was twenty-four and a graduate student in library sciences when her family first took her to see a psychiatrist. She had been divorced after a brief marriage. Although she had seemed flighty for some time, her behavior had become bizarre. She had begun to squander money foolishly, call people on the phone in the middle of the night, and disappear for days at a time. In the psychiatrist's office, she was obviously hyperactive and euphoric, with grandiose ideas. She spoke rapidly and jumped from subject to subject. The psychiatrist diagnosed her condition as a manic psychosis and recommended hospitalization, which Cathy refused. She did, however, agree to take medication and return to the psychiatrist for continuing treatment.

Although the psychiatrist prescribed lithium and increasing doses of antipsychotic medication, Cathey's behavior showed little change. She was dropped from classes but was able to get a job as a school librarian. Soon she began missing days at work, but a letter from the psychiatrist to the school principal indicating that she was under treatment for an emotional illness averted her being fired from the job. Similarly, a letter from the psychiatrist to the police extricated her from a shoplifting charge.

Cathy's case seemed to be so obviously a manic psychosis that the doctor never asked about her use of any chemicals. She had been drinking heavily for several years and more recently had begun to use marijuana liberally. One time the subject of drinking did arise, and the doctor advised her not to drink because the combination of alcohol and the antipsychotic medication was potentially dangerous; Cathy continued to drink anyway.

Cathy's flighty behavior changed little even with large doses of medication. However, she began to have days when she could hardly get out of bed in the morning, and a friend gave her a "picker–upper" in the form of amphetamines, a diet pill that this friend was taking. Cathy found these pills most helpful, and soon was on a fairly regular regimen of "booze, grass, and speed." She did not tell her doctor about this, and he continued to see her regularly and prescribe for her.

After many months, Cathy experienced a severe depression. The psychiatrist, unaware that she had been using amphetamines regularly but had not been able to get any for a few days and was experiencing the severe depression ("crashing") characteristic of amphetamine withdrawal, diagnosed the episode as the depressive phase of manic–depressive disease, and added antidepressants to her treatment.

For the next several years, Cathy continued to be treated with antipsychotic and antidepressant medication, and when she complained of insomnia, sedatives were prescribed. She continued to have wide mood swings with irrational behavior and was hospitalized three times for suicidal overdoses. During all this time, she continued to use alcohol, marijuana, amphetamines, and sleeping pills. Her close friends and some of her family knew of her heavy chemical indulgence, but their input was never sought, and Cathy did not volunteer the information.

After her third and very serious suicidal attempt Cathy's extensive use of alcohol and drugs came to light, and her psychiatrist referred her to our alcohol and chemical rehabilitation center. While in this center, all the drugs except lithium were discontinued, and Cathy was maintained on the lithium because of what appeared to be a *bona fide* manic–depressive illness for which lithium is specific.

Cathy completed a four-week course in the rehabilitation center and upon discharge was advised to continue her lithium. She became actively involved in Alcoholics Anonymous. I did not see her again until eight months later, at which time she told me that her recovery was beyond belief. "Imagine," she said, "I have not missed work for even a single day in eight months! That never happened to me before. I could not get through a single week without one or more absences previously."

I asked Cathy whom she was seeing for her lithium regulation, and she said, "No one. I am not taking lithium."

I told Cathy that I had advised her not to discontinue the lithium, to which she responded, "Look, doctor, I have been diagnosed as manic–depressive for twelve years; but I had been drinking and using chemicals for *fourteen* years. I may not even be manic–depressive. If I find out that I get depressed or high while I am sober, I will go back on lithium, but I owe it to myself to find out for certain."

At the time of this writing, Cathy is six years sober, is working regularly, and has not had any absences or disruptions because of either depression or mania. In a person who had not been symptom-free for even several days in twelve years, a six-year period of essentially excellent mental health is adequate grounds for assuming that what appeared to be a manic–depressive disorder was in reality behavior generated by alcohol, marijuana, amphetamines, and sedatives.

A similar diagnostic error can occur when heavy drinkers begin to hallucinate or have delusions of persecution. Unless the role of alcohol is known and the appropriate treatment instituted, these people may be treated for mental illness that they do not have.

Edward was in the army and was stationed in Korea. He had always been somewhat of a hell–raiser. Ed had been a heavy drinker since his late adolescence. He was raised in a wealthy family, and he had not been denied too many things. In the army, his drinking continued without much incident. He was not much different than many of his comrades who drank excessively.

One time on a four-day R & R leave in Japan, Ed drank extremely heavily and may have even used some drugs. When he returned to the base, he was "seeing things" and talking irrationally. He was seen by the army psychiatrist, who diagnosed him as "schizophrenic" and arranged for him to be returned to the United States.

During the next few days, Ed's thinking cleared considerably, but he was nevertheless sent home on a military plane in full restraints. He said that he had pleaded to be unshackled but was told that these were army regulations. His parents, who had been advised of Ed's return and the diagnosis of schizophrenia, arranged to have him transferred from a military hospital to a private hospital, where he was treated with insulin coma. Insulin coma is a treatment for schizophrenia that is no longer in use. It consisted of administering large doses of insulin so that the blood sugar dropped to the point where the brain was deprived of nutrients and the patient became unconscious for a period of time. It was held that a series of sixty such treatments could bring about a remission of the psychosis.

After being discharged from the hospital, Ed promptly resumed his heavy drinking and was soon rehospitalized. His diagnosis of schizophrenia followed him. As with most heavy drinkers who are forced to abstain, Ed did not sleep well in the hospital, and sedatives were prescribed. His doctor continued to prescribe the sedative after Ed was discharged from the hospital, and Ed used the sedative just as he did the alcohol—increasing the amount consumed until he achieved the desired effect.

During the next few years, Ed was in and out of mental hospitals. A review of the records from these hospitals revealed no reference to the excessive drinking on any of the admissions. The initial diagnosis of schizophrenia, made under the conditions of a military outpost, haunted Ed throughout his many hospitalizations. The alcoholism and subsequent drug addiction that was largely responsible for his behavior was never diagnosed and was never addressed in treatment.

Another case is that of a thirty-year-old young woman who

I was asked to see on consultation to evaluate her for possible electroshock treatment. The young woman was extremely depressed and was considered so severe a suicidal risk that she was ordered to have one of the nursing staff in constant attendance to prevent any sudden suicidal impulse.

During her interview, the patient, who is a registered nurse, described some situations within her marriage that were disturbing and also said she was terribly depressed about having been diagnosed several years earlier as an epileptic. Careful questioning regarding use of alcohol and drugs revealed that she indeed did drink frequently and also that she was taking Valium by prescription. The prescribing doctor had instructed her to take a maximum of 40 mg of Valium a day, but she reluctantly admitted that the amount was inadequate to "settle her nerves," and that she would take between 80 mg and 120 mg a day. She also said that the convulsive seizures that had led to her diagnosis of epilepsy had resulted when she tried to cut down the quantity of Valium she was taking.

It was thus evident that the diagnosis of epilepsy was incorrect and that this young woman had suffered withdrawal seizures. This meant that she did not have to look forward to a lifelong effort to control convulsive seizures and that she could be certain that if she stopped using alcohol and tranquilizers, she would not have any further seizures. It was also evident that her depression was essentially caused by her drinking and abuse of the prescribed drug.

After completing withdrawal from the medications, the young woman was admitted to a rehabilitation center, where she completed a successful course of therapy. She then joined Alcoholics Anonymous, has since continued her career in nursing, and her marriage has stabilized.

I have emphasized mood-altering chemicals as causes of emotional disorders because of their widespread use and the too frequent unawareness of this by both therapist and patient. However, medications that are not primarily mood-altering can also have marked psychological effects.

The depression–producing effects of reserpine and decongestants have already been noted. Other medications that are used to treat blood pressure can have similar effects. Birth-control pills have been implicated in causing depression, as have some anti-inflammatory drugs, such as those used for pain relief in arthritis. Corticosteroids may produce mood changes, both "highs" and "lows." Patients with heart disease who receive digitalis preparations may build up too-high blood levels of this medication, and the only symptom of this may be depression or confusion. Mistaking this mood or mental change for a psychotic disorder can result in even fatal digitalis poisoning. Elderly patients may be sensitive to the antispasmodics frequently prescribed for gastrointestinal disorders and may develop severe confusion and even hallucinations. I recall an elderly woman who developed visual hallucinations as a result of the eye drops she received while undergoing an eye examination.

Pierce was a sixty-two-year-old retired millworker, who was admitted psychiatrically because he had been depressed about a month. His appetite had fallen off, and he was not sleeping well. He had retired from the mill at age fifty-nine but had always managed to keep himself busy around the house. He did not drink to excess.

Prior to his retirement, Pierce had developed shortness of breath on exertion and was found to have heart disease. In fact, the heart disease led to his early retirement. He was treated by an elderly doctor who had been the family physician for several generations. He saw his doctor once a month.

When Pierce began developing depressive symptoms, his doctor prescribed antidepressant medication. Instead of improving, Pierce's condition worsened, and he had several episodes of confusion. His doctor then called a psychiatrist to have him admitted to the psychiatric unit.

Pierce resisted admission because of unpleasant associations and on several occasions Pierce had had to act as the responsible with mental hospitals. Pierce's brother had been mentally ill, and on several occasions Pierce had had to act as the responsible family member to have him committed. The brother eventually committed suicide. Pierce's reluctance to enter a mental hospital was understandable. Only after persistent pressure by his wife and children and under threat of commitment did Pierce sign himself into the hospital, but not before he vowed to disown all his children for coercing him to do so.

On the day following admission to the hospital, an electro-cardiogram was done, which revealed signs of digitalis toxicity. Pierce had been taking the same dose of digitalis daily for several years. The psychiatrist consulted an internist, and after appropriate management of the digitalis toxicity, Pierce's mental status improved dramatically without any specific psychiatric treatment.

The reason Pierce had developed digitalis poisoning was never elucidated. However, digitalis is a drug that, for all its value, can produce toxic effects when changes occur in the body that cause a higher blood level of the drug or an increased sensitivity to the drug's effects. This can occur even if the dosage is not increased. Sometimes the only symptoms of toxicity are mental, and the patient, like Pierce, may be misdiagnosed as having a functional psychiatric illness.

Patients who are being treated by more than one physician may be taking medication prescribed by each doctor without the other knowing what else has been prescribed; the interaction between two medications can produce mental changes in some cases. Over-the-counter medications should not be considered to be without risk. Many can produce the symptoms just described.

Awareness of the possibility of mental or mood changes resulting from the use of alcohol or drugs can help both the patient and physician to properly evaluate symptoms. A logical first step would be to eliminate all use of alcohol or drugs (when feasible) for a period of at least a month, and observe the patient's course. Physicians often suggest that people who develop skin rashes of undetermined origin eliminate certain foods for a period of time to see whether the rash improves. It is difficult to understand why the same approach is not used more often with alcohol. If the patient cannot abstain from alcohol for at least this period of time, there is considerable reason to believe that an addiction problem exists. Patients with symptoms of depression who are being treated with a particular drug, such as those used for high blood pressure, can often be switched to a different drug for treatment of this condition.

Western civilization is not only overdosed with alcohol but also expects miraculous treatment with some wonder drug for all discomforts. While medications are often a lifesaving blessing, any chemical that is biologically active can be indiscriminate in its effects. Failure to recognize this may lead to mistaken psychiatric diagnosis and inappropriate treatment.

10

Brain Disorders

A fifty-seven-year-old man was admitted to the psychiatric hospital because of a "psychosis." On initial examination, the patient's response to questions were nonsensical; for example, the answer had no relevance to the question. Example: Q: "Hello, my name is Dr. Twerski. Please tell me your name." A: "That's right. I didn't do anything wrong. I am all right."

Prior to admission to the hospital, this patient had undergone a physical examination in the emergency room, which was completely normal with one exception. The only abnormality was that his conversation was incoherent and irrelevant. He had a tendency to repeat the same phrase over and over.

A phone call to the patient's wife elicited the following information. The patient had been in good health and had gone to work that day as he had for the past twenty-one years. He was not a drinker and was not on medication. In the afternoon, she had received a call from his employer that the patient had "gone crazy" and was "talking out of his head." He was taken to a hospital emergency room and was thereafter admitted to the psychiatric hospital for "psychosis."

Severe mental illnesses rarely strike suddenly in a person who has been mentally stable. The abrupt onset of the patient's abnormal behavior was strongly suggestive of a stroke, and X-rays done following injection of dye into the blood vessels leading to the brain (angiogram) demonstrated that the patient had indeed suffered a stroke. This particular patient had an unusual type of stroke, with no paralysis or weakness of either arm or leg. The only area of the brain that was affected by the sudden blockage of a blood vessel was the area that controls comprehension of speech; hence, the patient's responses were nonsensical because he was unable to understand what was said to him. Absence of the usual facial or limb paralysis accompanying a typical stroke obscured the correct diagnosis and resulted in the patient being considered "crazy."

A thirty-two-year-old college chemistry instructor was admitted to a psychiatric unit because he had become very withdrawn and had been failing to show up for classes. Ten years earlier, he had been diagnosed as epileptic and had been taking anticonvulsant medication. A neurological examination shortly after admission suggested a brain tumor, and a brain scan confirmed the presence of a very large growth inside the brain.

Annette was twenty-six when she had her first child. She and Fred had both looked forward to the baby as the solution to their marital problems. Early in the marriage, they had both accused each other of being self-centered, and the two sets of in-laws had helped fuel the flames. When Annette became pregnant, there was initial concern about a child coming into a marriage whose survival was in doubt. However, because termination of the pregnancy was ruled out on religious grounds, Annette and Fred decided to make every effort to save the marriage, especially because they would now both have an interest in someone other than themselves who belonged to both of them.

About six weeks after the baby's birth, Annette began to have crying spells, to lose her appetite, and to sleep poorly. She said she felt no love for the baby and was unable to care for her. The baby was taken to Annette's parents' home for care, and Annette was seen by a psychiatrist, who diagnosed her condition as a post-partum depression. Annette was hospitalized for several weeks and was then treated as an outpatient. She made a good recovery and resumed care of her child.

When the baby was about a year old, Annette began complaining of severe headaches. She was seen in an emergency room, where a brief physical examination failed to find a cause. She told the emergency room doctor that she was taking medication for her depression, and he advised her that the headaches were emotional in origin and related to the depression. He suggested she take some aspirin and return to her psychiatrist.

Annette made two more visits to the emergency room the same week because of severe headaches, and each time was told the same thing. She then went to a second hospital emergency room, where she was examined. A psychiatrist was called in for consultation and found that she was withdrawn and had been crying; he concurred that the patient was depressed and should continue to see her own psychiatrist.

Several days later, Annette was back in the emergency room complaining of severe headache, nausea, and vomiting. A young resident was on duty, and Annette did not tell him about her psychiatric problem. After examining her, the resident did a spinal tap, which confirmed his diagnosis of viral meningitis, and Annette was hospitalized in the general hospital, where she had an uneventful recovery.

These are several examples of what can happen within the brain that can give an impression of mental illness.

Because the brain is the organ that is the origin of all thought and feeling processes and consequently all behavior, anything that causes impairment of brain function is very likely to bring about behavioral changes. Such behavior may very well be mistaken for one of the many forms of mental illness. Often the brain disease is treatable, but if the disease is not correctly diagnosed, the patient may be treated psychiatrically while a disease progressively destroys more brain tissue.

Some conditions that affect the brain are so rare (porphyria, Wilson's disease) that a psychiatrist may go through a lifetime of practice without seeing a single case of a particular disease. This makes it less likely that the doctor will consider the rare diseases as possible diagnoses. As mentioned earlier, this is no justification and of no comfort whatever to the one patient who does have the unusual disease.

Epilepsy is a disease that occurs frequently and is most often manifested by episodic, violent body movements. One type of seizure disorder, psychomotor epilepsy, is not at all uncommon; and because it occurs without body convulsions and its primary symptoms may all be behavioral, psychomotor epilepsy can be mistaken for a psychiatric disorder. Psychomotor epilepsy may manifest itself in mood swings and may be mistaken for manic–depressive disease. It may cause angry outbursts and may be diagnosed as "aggressive personality." If hallucinations occur, it may be considered to be schizophrenia. The correct diagnosis is of utmost importance, because recent advances have been achieved in the treatment of psychomotor epilepsy, but application of the appropriate treatment presupposes the correct diagnosis.[1]

Roseanne had been a difficult child, and her adolescence was particularly stormy. She was in frequent disagreement with her parents, whose efforts to control her impulsiveness were futile. When she did not get what she wanted, she would often sulk and withdraw to her room, although at times she would react by shouting and screaming. At other times she would leave home for a night to stay at a girlfriend's home.

Roseanne's parents indulged her behavior because they felt responsible for the way she acted. When Roseanne was five, her mother suffered a "nervous breakdown" that necessitated her being hospitalized for several months. During this period of time, Roseanne had been cared for by friends and relatives. She was, of course, too young to understand that her mother was ill, and she had not been permitted to visit her mother until a few

[1]D. F. Benson and D. Blumer, *Psychiatric Aspects of Neurologic Disease*, (New York: Grune and Shatter. 1975), 171–198; E. H. Reynolds and M. R. Trimble, *Epilepsy and Psychiatry*, (New York: Churchil Livinstone, 1981), 131–137.

weeks before her discharge from the hospital. The parents believed that Roseanne had felt deserted by her mother, who in turn felt guilty that she had "let herself go" to the point of becoming severely mentally ill. The father, on the other hand, took himself to task for what he considered to be his contribution to his wife's mental problems. Roseanne's parents appeared to reinforce each other's guilt, and both felt that they had deprived the child of parental attention at a crucial phase of her development and that they therefore had to bear the consequences of their dereliction.

After Roseanne turned eighteen, her behavior changed markedly, manifested by episodes of intense rage and outbursts of violence during which she would break things and occasionally physically attack her parents. Sometimes it appeared that she was grossly overreacting to some trivial frustration, and at other times, no evident precipitating event could account for her reaction. These episodes lasted but a few minutes, and immediately afterward Roseanne would appear confused, exhausted, and extremely remorseful.

Roseanne's parents had hesitated to take her to a psychiatrist. They believed that because they had brought the problem about, they had to suffer in silence and deal with it as best they could. The mother in particular felt that she had been stigmatized as a mental patient and did not want Roseanne to carry that label. One time, however, Roseanne became so violent that the parents had no option other than to have her taken to a hospital emergency room, where she was examined and admitted to the psychiatric service.

The psychiatric and psychological evaluations confirmed what Roseanne's parents had already assumed; namely, that Roseanne was immature and very insecure. She had never resolved the feeling that her mother had abandoned her, and her being shifted among several homes during her mother's hospitalization had indeed left her with the feeling that she was undesirable and was being rejected by everyone. Therapy would be long and arduous. The parents would have to anticipate more violent episodes until the psychological problems could be resolved. If the parents felt they were unable to cope with her violence, Roseanne would have to be treated as an inpatient, but prolonged hospitalization would likely reinforce her feelings of rejection.

Almost as an afterthought, the psychiatrist requested consultation with a neurologist. Although the examination was essentially normal, the neurologist thought he detected "soft signs," or subtle findings that might be but were not necessarily abnormal. A brain scan was performed, which was normal, but the electroencephalogram showed some changes that were compatible with although not diagnostic of a convulsive disorder: psychomotor epilepsy.

The EEG findings led to rethinking of the symptoms: brief outbursts, sometimes without provocation, followed by weakness and confusion. The doctors decided to institute treatment with anticonvulsant medications.

Roseanne had no further violent outbursts. Her course in psychotherapy was able to continue satisfactorily.

Multiple sclerosis is a disease that is characterized by episodes of remission during which the patient may appear completely normal. Because various parts of the brain and spinal cord may be alternately affected, symptoms may not be consistent. A patient may have temporary loss of vision at one time and paralysis of arm or leg another time; yet a doctor may not find anything during an examination.

Understandably, a person who has even a temporary loss of vision, paralysis of an arm or leg, or loss of equilibrium can become very upset. The patient may become depressed or may be very anxious because of what is happening to him. The anxiety and depression may persist long after the physical symptoms have passed. If the examining physician sees only the emotional symptoms and finds no physical disturbance, all too likely the patient may be diagnosed as neurotic.

The case of the chemistry instructor cited in the beginning of this chapter demonstrates yet another point. That patient had developed convulsive seizures at age twenty-two and at that time had undergone a neurologic examination that was reported as negative, with a diagnosis of epilepsy. The patient continued to take anticonvulsant medication for ten years without having a neurologic reexamination. Although the first seizure was undoubtedly caused by the tumor, the tumor was at that time so small that it could not be detected by examination or tests. However, somewhere along the ten-year course, a reexamination would have revealed the tumor before it had grown large enough to threaten the patient's life. At that point, surgery might well have been successful.

This case indicates that a negative medical workup when the patient presents symptoms may not necessarily be conclusive. If the mental symptoms persist, repeated examinations may be necessary.

Too often, once patients acquire a psychiatric diagnosis, labels are apt to follow them throughout their lifetimes. If subsequently the treatment of these patients is taken over by other therapists, the latter may assume that the diagnosis of depression, schizophrenia, hysteria, or anxiety neurosis is correct and may not press for a complete medical evaluation. Certainly therapists who see patients for a prolonged period of time for what they have assumed to be "functional" mental illness, are not likely to change their orientation midway. Indeed, if therapists are seeing the patients regularly, physical symptoms that have been persistent or even outward changes in appearance that have developed gradually might not arouse suspicion of an underlying medical problem.

The "labeling" phenomenon obviously applies to all kinds of medical disorders and not only to brain changes. Some people acquire a label of hypochondriac or "crank" because they consistently complain about varying symptoms for which the doctor can never discover a physical cause. Like the boy who cried "wolf," they may get into trouble when a serious physical problem does arise.

A sixty-year-old woman was referred by a state hospital physician to our hospital for a medical evaluation. She had admitted herself voluntarily to the state hospital on the insistence of her family physician, who had threatened that if she did not do so he would have her committed. She had been depressed for many years, and when she began having difficulty sleeping, her doctor told her that she had to deal with the depression once and for all and that he was tired of all her "bellyaching." Her loss of sleep was primarily caused by a persistent cough that had not been relieved by cough medication and that her doctor had diagnosed as "a neurotic cough."

An alert physician at the state hospital thought that the patient might have some chest disease that needed further evaluation. Indeed, she was found to have a collection of fluid in her lungs because of cancer. Earlier diagnosis conceivably could have saved this woman's life, but her label of hypochondriasis, which she might have justly acquired over the years, had led her physician astray.

Returning to brain disorders, the suspicion of possible brain involvement must always be maintained. Minute brain-tissue changes, too tiny to be detected by any tests currently available, may cause subtle changes in mental acuity of which only the patients may be aware. They may notice that they cannot think as clearly as they used to, cannot perform rather simple mathematical calculations, and may have developed memory impairment very different from the usual "I can no longer recall people's names." The patients may be very vague about their symptoms and may be hesitant to let on that something is happening, but they are apt to react to their perception of impaired mental function with a rather marked personality change. They may become very depressed or very irritable, critical, and argumentative. In certain brain diseases such as tumor, the growth itself may be responsible for personality changes, but

sometimes the personality symptoms are the patients' reaction to
a subtle deterioration. Because examination in the early stages
may not reveal any tissue disease, a psychiatric diagnosis is
likely to be made. This move cannot be criticized, because
doctors can go only by what they see. However, although
psychiatric therapy may be initiated, somewhere along the
line the brain should be reevaluated, which might reveal a
physical problem early enough to permit effective treatment.

11

Sundry Others

Donna was a nineteen-year-old who was referred for a psychiatric admission after having been examined in another hospital emergency room and being diagnosed as having "catatonic schizoprenia," a type of psychosis where the patient is frequently mute and motionless. At our emergency room, she was again examined and indeed found to be mute; she did not talk but responded to questions with head gestures only.

Donna's father had accompanied her to the hospital but could not give much information about her. He said that he was divorced from Donna's mother and was now remarried for the third time. He had very little contact with Donna, who had alternately lived with her mother and her maternal grandmother. The father described Donna's mother's home as very unstable, because the mother had numerous liaisons with various men. The grandmother, on the other hand, was overly strict, and Donna had not adjusted in either household. She had taken off with friends several times, but because of the lack of a steady home, no one knew she had gone.

The absence of any stability in Donna's life was certainly conducive to the development of an emotional disorder. Being shunted from place to place with no real investment in her welfare by either parent and no demonstration of being wanted by anyone might be expected to result in schizophrenia. Donna was thus admitted to the psychiatric service.

On the following morning, the routine laboratory studies revealed Donna to be in severe kidney failure and as a result of which she had a very low level of calcium in her blood. The latter causes severe muscular spasms, particularly of the jaw muscles. The reason this young woman did not talk was not because she was catatonic but simply because *she could not physically open her mouth* because of the spastic muscles that clamped her jaws shut. After treatment on the artificial kidney, she was no longer "mute" or catatonic.

Other disturbances in the blood chemistries can present misleading pictures. Patients who are on diuretic medication, usually for treatment of high blood pressure or heart disease, may lose excessive amounts of sodium and/or potassium. Low blood levels of these two elements can produce varying psychiatric symptoms, which can easily be mistaken for psychoses.[1] Mineral losses can also occur with some gastrointestinal diseases in which there is protracted vomiting and diarrhea. Inadequate function of the adrenal glands (Addison's disease) may also produce this condition and has been known to manifest itself with psychotic delusions.[2]

Elevation of the blood calcium, which can occur in several diseases, can give rise to quite severe mental symptoms, which disappear when the blood level returns to normal.[3]

Although rather infrequent, lead, mercury, and other metal poisonings can occur, and the most prominent symptoms in these cases may be mental.[4]

Claire was forty-two years old and was admitted to the

[1]G. M. Burnell and T. A. Foster, "Psychosis With Low Sodium Syndrome," *American Journal of Psychiatry*, 128, 10 (1974): 133–134; M. Gehi, R. Rosenthal, N. Fizehe, L. Crowe, and W. Webb, "Psychiatric Manifestations of Hyponatremia," *Psychosomatics*, 22:9 (1981), 739–743.
[2]M. L. Koran and D. A. Hamburg, "Psychophysiological Endocrine Disorders," *Comprehensive Textbook of Psychiatry I*, second edition. A. M. Freedman, H. I. Kaplan, and B. J. Sadoh, eds. (Baltimore, Md.: William and Wilkins, 1975), 1673–1684.
[3]W. L. Webb, and Gehi, "Disorders of Fluid and Electrolyte Balance," *Psychiatric Presentation of Medical Illness*, R. W. Hall, editor, (New York: Spectrum Publications, 1980), 259–299.
[4]N. Edwards, "Mental Disturbances Related to Metals," *Psychiatric Presentation of Medical Illness*, Hall, ed., (New York: Spectrum Publications, 1980), 283–308.

psychiatric unit of a general hospital because of severe depression. Several months prior to her admission, her only son had married and moved out of the house. Claire, too, was an only child. Her husband was often away from home for days on business trips, and after the son's marriage, Claire often stayed with her parents. It was assumed that Claire's depression was brought on by her loneliness.

Claire's depression was characterized by an unusual manifestation of anger, which was totally unlike her previous personality. When her parents came in to visit, she would swear at them and order them out. She used obscene language, which was completely out of character. Physical examination and routine admission laboratory studies were negative. She was diagnosed as an acute severe depression, and because of the severity of the symptoms, electroshock was recommended.

Claire's husband was hesitant to consent to electroshock, and she was treated with antipsychotic drugs while several consultants were called in. She then became severely confused and disoriented. Doctors assumed that she had a reaction to the medications, and these were discontinued. She then developed a fever and a rash. Reevaluation by the medical consultants and special tests confirmed the diagnosis of systemic lupus erythematosus, a disease that affects many systems, including the brain. Claire was treated with corticosteroids, and her mental symptoms cleared completely.

Cases of lupus erythematosus with mental symptoms appear in the medical literature.[5] Generally the mental symptoms appear in the course of disease that has been diagnosed by other manifestations, but sometimes the mental features are the only symptoms, making the correct diagnosis difficult.[6] This is also true of *periarteritis nodosa,* a disease that primarily involves

---

[5]J. A. Denburg, *et al.,* "Pathogenesis of Neurosystematic Lupus," *Canadian Medical Association Journal* 128 (3) (1983): 257–260.

[6]D. M. MacNeill, *et. al.,* "Psychiatric Problems in Systemic Lupus Erythematosus," *British Journal of Psychiatry* 128 (1976): 442–455.

blood vessels and muscles but which can produce mental symptoms.

Psychiatric symptoms may occur several weeks following a viral infection, where the patient had the usual "cold" symptoms with severe headache and stiff neck. This may represent a mild viral encephalitis, wherein the virus affects the brain.[7] Although there may not be any specific treatment for the virus infection, and the patient may actually have to be treated just as though this were a functional mental illness, the correct diagnosis is nevertheless of utmost importance.

Patients who recover from a severe mental illness are always concerned about their prognosis. Is this likely to happen again? Is there anything I can do to prevent a recurrence? Is this hereditary, which can be passed down to my children? If the diagnosis is functional mental illness whose cause is at best conjectural, the doctor can tell the patient relatively little that is reassuring. If the mental symptoms are indeed secondary to a viral encephalitis or other brain-tissue disease, the patient can be assured that his mind is functionally sound.

I have had personal experience with several cases where patients were brought to the hospital from the local bus station with frank psychoses. All were similar in that they had developed delusions of persecution, believing that other passengers in the bus were out to get them or that people outside of the bus were trying to get in to harm them. All these patients were enroute from the West Coast and had developed their symptoms shortly before approaching Pittsburgh. In all cases, contact with the families revealed no previous history of mental disorder, and all these patients were perfectly normal after one or two days in the hospital. They recalled their experiences with bewilderment about why they had had such "crazy" thoughts.

[7] J. Himmelhoch, J. Pincus, G. Tucker, and T. Detre, "Subacute Encephalitis: Behavioral and Neurological Aspects," *British Journal of Psychiatry* 116 (1970): 531–538; L. G. Wilson, "Viral Encelphalopathy Mimicking Functional Psychoses," *Americal Journal of Psychiatry* 134 (1976): 165–170.

The mystery is explained by the fact that these people were light sleepers and had been unable to sleep at all on the bus. By the time they had reached Pittsburgh from California, the deprivation of sleep was sufficient to throw them into acute psychotic reactions.

Sleep deprivation has been known to produce mental symptoms. Obviously, circumstances other than long bus rides can result in prolonged sleep deprivation, and before concluding that persecutory delusions and hallucinations are indicative of paranoid schizophrenia, inquiry should be made into such circumstances. An acute onset of psychotic ideation in a person previously felt to be psychologically stable should make the therapist consider sleep deprivation as a possible cause.

Mental symptoms resulting from sleep deprivation may not be all that uncommon. In some cases the true facts are simply not recognized.

Oliver was a seventy-one-year-old married man, who had retired from his job as a bookkeeper at sixty-five. He had made a fair adjustment to retirement, occupying himself with the management of two small properties he had acquired, taking care of the maintenance and necessary repairs, as well as managing the family finances. Over a period of several weeks, he began showing significant mental changes. His memory deteriorated rapidly, and the tenants complained to his wife that he would go back several times the same day for the same things. His mathematical acuity changed drastically, and he made gross errors in the checking account. He also developed a shuffling gait, and his interest in things dropped significantly.

Oliver was examined by his family physician. He had always enjoyed good health, and except for a mild elevation of the blood pressure, his physical workup showed nothing wrong. He had symptoms of prostate trouble for the past several years and would awaken three to four times a night to urinate. However, he had refused prostate surgery. The doctor told the family that Oliver had begun to undergo senile changes and that there was no specific treatment for this.

Things went on without much change for about six months. Oliver had some days that were better, when he seemed to be his "old self," alert, quite keen, and ready and willing to do things. Most days, however, he appeared confused, depressed, and withdrawn. The doctor said these variations were caused by changes in blood circulation.

One morning Oliver was unable to get out of bed and was unable to speak. His wife called the physician, who said that this appeared to be a stroke, and arranged for prompt hospitalization. Within several hours, however, his speech returned to normal. A series of tests were done, and it was determined that Oliver had experienced a transient ischemic attack, or a brief deprivation of blood flow to the brain. His blood chemistries were all normal.

While in the hospital Oliver wet the bed on several occasions. A urologist was consulted, and after some urging, Oliver agreed to undergo prostate surgery. Following the surgery, he had an uneventful recovery.

After returning home, everyone was surprised to note the marked improvement in Oliver's mental status. He no longer had any days of confusion and depression. His memory appeared to be intact, and his mathematical calculations were once again precise.

The mystery of Oliver's difficulty and recovery then became clear. Not only had Oliver been suffering from repeated interruptions of his sleep because of the prostate problem and the need to go to the bathroom several times during the night, but after an embarrassing episode when he wet the bed at home one night, he would fight sleep because he was afraid this might happen again. He thus "cat napped" throughout the night, and the mental symptoms he was manifesting were caused by sleep deprivation. Those nights that he had better sleep were followed by days on which his mental status was much better. After the prostate surgery corrected the problem and he returned to normal sleep, his mental symptoms cleared completely.

Under normal circumstances, we are bombarded by sensory stimuli from all sides. We generally hear various sounds and look at different things. As we move about, we come into tactile contact with many things. If there is a drastic reduction in the stimuli impacting on a person, hallucinations may develop.

This is not an uncommon occurrence in patients who have undergone eye surgery and who have both eyes patched. If the patient is also bedfast, visual stimuli are completely eliminated and tactile contact is sharply reduced. These patients are apt to hallucinate, and the hallucinations may lead to delusions. If the patient is also hard of hearing, the sensory deprivation may be nearly complete. Ophthalmologists therefore instruct nurses and family members to be in frequent contact with patients, to talk to them, and to touch them frequently.

Outside of the hospital, the same phenomenon can occur in people who are housebound and who develop severe impairment of vision and hearing loss. Sensory deprivation psychoses in these people may actually be prevented by providing more frequent human contact, with visits by family and neighbors, and by getting the person out of the house as often as is feasible.

Although people generally assume hallucinations to be an indication of "craziness," it is universally accepted that hallucinations during sleep, or in other words dreams, are perfectly normal. However, hallucinations also can occur in the "twilight" phase between sleep and awakening, and although they may be very frightening, they are not abnormal phenomena.

A twenty-three-year-old man came for psychiatric consultation because he was certain he was "cracking up." While lying in bed one day, he saw the wall before him open up, and a hand holding a pitcher was extended. After pouring out some liquid, the hand retracted and the wall closed. He wanted to go over and check out this vision but felt himself totally immobile as though he were paralyzed. He became very anxious and broke out in a cold sweat. A few minutes later, he was able to get up and check both the wall and floor, finding no sign of any opening in the wall nor any liquid on the floor. He was then convinced that he must be losing his mind.

Hallucinations such as these, which are very vivid, may occur as one is falling asleep (hypnogogic) or as one is emerging from sleep (hypnopompic). They may occur in people who have no mental abnormality.

People who have an unusual sensitivity regarding psychiatric problems, for example someone who has had a case of mental illness in a family member, may react with considerable anxiety to any strange experience or feeling. The common *deja vu* phenomenon, where people have an eerie feeling that they have already experienced a particular scene or been in a place when they are actually there for the first time, may frighten people who have had say, a psychotic parent. Similarly, feelings of clairvoyance may be very threatening. Thinking of a tune and then hearing someone begin to hum it may make people consider whether someone is reading their mind or controlling their thoughts. These and other mental phenomena that are not indicative of mental illness are described in a delightful book, Your Normal Mind.[8]

Thus, here are some cases in which simple reassurance provided by an authoritative person may thwart the development of severe anxiety or other emotional distress.

[8]L. Pollack, *Your Normal Mind*, (New York: Wilfred Funk, 1951).

12

In Later Years

A great deal is heard about the health and social problems of the elderly and rightly so. The prolongation of life made possible by medical progress has resulted in the emergence of new problems unique to older people. Special consideration of the the health conditions of the elderly is of particular importance in diagnosing mental illness.

Senility, or what is known medically as Alzheimer's disease, is unfortunately all too common in advanced age. The cause of Alzheimer's disease is as yet unknown, although most doctors have assumed that old brain cells simply wear out. However, definite chemical changes occur in brain cells in Alzheimer's disease, and this condition can also occur in people age forty or fifty, to whom the "worn out" theory does not apply.

The symptoms of senility are well-known. People exhibit progressive confusion, loss of memory, and impaired judgment —all ultimately resulting in the inability to function independently. General physical health is often quite good. In advanced stages, the mental deterioration may be so severe that people can no longer function without constant supervision; this often means custodial care in some institution for the aged. At this point in time, there is no known treatment for Alzheimer's disease.

Because no laboratory test can confirm the diagnosis of Alzheimer's, the diagnosis is generally made on the basis of observed signs and symptoms. These can be misleading. Because the diagnosis is essentially that of an untreatable condition, great care must be taken that a patient is not erroneously given a prognosis of hopelessness.

Some elderly people may have lost some brain cells but are still able to function normally as long as all the remaining cells are functioning at full capacity. Some "wear and tear" conditions are common to the elderly, and they can result in very marginal functioning. Younger people have a kind of "reserve capacity" that older people lack, and relatively small changes in health that would be insignificant in younger people can have major effects in the elderly.

Some elderly people have inefficient circulatory systems. Just as we may find a buildup of deposits of precipitates and sludge in old plumbing that reduces the lumen of the pipes, so we often find narrowing of the blood vessels because of arteriosclerosis in the elderly, which compromises the flow of blood, particularly to the brain. Just enough blood may be getting through to permit normal brain activity and normal functioning. Anything that even minimally affects the blood flow to the brain or the ability of the blood that does get through to deliver enough oxygen to the brain cells can therefore be sufficient to push the older person "over the edge."

A younger person whose blood count should be between 12 grams and 14 grams hemoglobin percent can still have a good mental functioning even with an anemia of 9 grams to 10 grams percent. In the older person whose mental function depends on all remaining viable cells getting all the oxygen they need, this degree of anemia can be enough to cause some symptoms of senility. Less than optimum heart function can also reduce the flow of blood to the brain. Chronic lung diseases, such as emphysema, that impair full oxygenation may contribute to mental changes. Chronic infection or even mild metabolic changes can have similar effects. Some older people may have more than one of these factors.

A seventy-eight-year-old man was admitted to the psychiatric hospital with a diagnosis of senility. He had been failing mentally for the past year. Medical evaluation revealed a mild anemia and a decrease in kidney function. Further examination showed that enlargement of the prostate gland had caused urinary obstruction and impairment of kidney function. The patient underwent surgery for removal of the prostatic obstruction. His kidney function improved significantly, and his mental status cleared, with much less confusion and better memory. He returned to his daughter's home, where he lived very happily for five years, dying peacefully in his sleep. If the correctible urinary problem had not been detected, this patient would have spent his last years (months?) in an institution, labeled as "senile."

A seventy-two-year-old woman was admitted to the psychiatric hospital because of "depression and senility." She had been under a doctor's care for heart disease but in recent weeks had been very cranky and forgetful and was unable to sleep through the night. Medical evaluation on the psychiatric unit revealed her to be suffering from moderate congestive heart failure. She responded well to the treatment of the heart disease, whereupon her mental symptoms disappeared.

Another problem that may be unique to the elderly is demonstrated by the case of a seventy-year-old retired chemistry professor, who was admitted to the hospital with delerium tremens, a very severe and dangerous withdrawal reaction from too much drinking. For several days, he was completely incoherent and was constantly hallucinating. After the delerium subsided, his memory was impaired and he was grossly confused. He had no concept of either time or place. As a result of the extensive drinking, he had also suffered damage to the nerves of his legs, and he was unable to walk or even stand.

After several weeks of treatment in the hospital with intensive vitamins, his memory impairment and confusion remained unchanged. A CAT scan of the brain showed that he had indeed suffered loss of some brain tissue. The many years of heavy drinking, perhaps combined with some senile changes, had taken their toll, and the patient was beyond recovery. The family was therefore advised to look for a facility that could care for him, which meant either a nursing home or the state hospital.

Eventually, procedures for commitment to the state hospital were initiated, but these were fraught with technical delays. However, during the waiting period, the patient's mental function began to improve, and by the time the day of the court hearing for commitment to the state hospital arrived, he had improved so much that the commitment hearing was canceled. The patient's mental status continued to improve sufficiently for admission to an alcohol rehabilitation center. He subsequently returned to his family and functioned at a high level of mental alertness, often assisting with the recovery of other elderly alcoholics, until he died of a heart attack five years later.

This case demonstrates a most important point. The time necessary for an older person to recover from reversible brain damage is apt to be much longer than that of a younger person. In the latter, persistent confusion for two to three weeks after recovery from the acute illness may well mean the patient has suffered permanent brain damage. In the older person, the period for restoration to normal may be six to eight weeks or longer, and diagnosing permanent brain damage in a lesser period may be erroneous.

The reason this is so important is that Medicare regulations will not authorize hospitalization for eight weeks following treatment of an acute illness for "observation." If patients are too confused to be cared for at home, they may be placed in a nursing home or state hospital. While some nursing homes and state hospitals are excellent, some lack adequate staff to do more than provide minimal care. A confused patient who wanders around and gets into trouble may be managed with sedatives and tranquilizers. If the patient has a reversible mental condition, the persistent administration of sedatives and tranquilizers may actually prevent the return of normal mental function.

It is tragic enough to have so many people with true Alzhiemer's disease for whom there is nothing one can do other than provide them with nutrition and supervision so that they do not harm themselves. It is infinitely more tragic to have a person who could potentially recover and lead an active life become a nonproductive institutional inmate only because no adequate evaluation can be provided.

Another factor may result in premature or erroneous diagnosis of senility. As mentioned, an older person's brain circulation may be marginal. A small drop in blood pressure, occurring either spontaneously or often as a result of a medication that the patients may be taking, may be enough to cause a temporary lack of blood supply to the brain. The patients may become suddenly bewildered and confused. They may not know where they are or may fail to recognize their families. They may wander away from the house and "come to" several blocks away. Such an episode is likely to be transient, and normal mental function returns within a few minutes. These are referred to as "transient ischemic attacks."

Understandably, the families may become alarmed and may take the patients to the doctor or to a hospital emergency room. Often nothing can be found on medical evaluation; at other times, something is detected in the respiratory, circulatory, or some other system. The doctor may recommend hospitalization for a more comprehensive medical workup.

Hospitalizing elderly people who are functioning marginally may present a problem. Anyone who has spent a night away from home may recall a moment of confusion on awakening in an unfamiliar place and then quickly reorienting oneself to the new environment. Elderly people may not be able to do this. Having been accustomed for the past thirty years to get up in the morning, walk ten feet down the corridor and turn left into the bathroom, they are apt to do the same thing when they wake up in the hospital, especially if their brains have been rendered groggy by the sedation they were given the previous night. However, the left turn now places them not in their bathroom, but in the room of another patient, who screams with fright at this intruder. A nurse and several nurses' aides come running and try to take the intruder out of the room. The patient is too confused to understand what is happening, and so resists their efforts. They begin using more brawn than brain, which agitates the patient and he fights back. The patient is eventually placed back in bed, perhaps with a waistband restraint to keep him in place, and the house doctor orders some tranquilizer to keep the patient quiet. If the patient struggles against the waist band, he may receive yet more sedation. He now feels imprisoned, which causes more agitation, and because he is too sedated to be able to think clearly, a vicious cycle may result, which may terminate in a long psychiatric hospitalization and possibly permanent institutionalization.

Every effort should therefore be made to keep elderly people within a familiar environment. Hospitalization should be used only when absolutely essential, and if possible, people familiar to the patients should be with them for as much time as is feasible, day and night.

Recently, articles in the medical literature have pointed out that in the elderly, depression can easily be mistaken for senility.[1] Even psychological tests and CAT scans may not be able to distinguish the two, and many psychiatrists feel that if there is any doubt whatever, patients should be given a trial of antidepressant therapy. Because the elderly are sensitive to medications and are especially prone to have unwanted side effects, the initial dosage must be low, and increases made gradually. This,

[1] D. F. Benson and D. Blumer, *Psychiatric Aspects of Alzheimer's Disease*, (New York: Grune and Stratton. 1975), 99–120.

of course, requires an extended period of time, and for reasons cited above, hospitalizing patients for this period of time, even if feasible, may be counterproductive.

The appropriate treatment of elderly patients who show signs of mental deterioration therefore requires careful planning and close cooperation between the physician, family, and available resources such as home health care providers. Only in this way can the tragedy of mistaken diagnosis and treatment be avoided.[2]

[2]C. M. Gaitz, "Identifying and Treating Depression in an Older Patient," *Geriatrics* 38 (2) (1983): 42–46; A. Comfort, *Practice of Geriatric Psychiatry*, (New York: Elseven/New Holland, 1980).

13

On the
Other Hand . . .

Although my intent in this book is to stress the importance of avoiding erroneous diagnoses of mental illness, it is of equal importance to avoid an error in the reverse direction, such as diagnosing and treating a physical condition when the true problem is of an emotional nature.

Diagnosing human ills is akin to walking a tightrope. If one leans too far to one side, the results can be disastrous; but if one attempts to overcorrect by leaning too far to the other side, the consequences are no better. There is a narrow range between whose borders one must walk for safe arrival.

Depressive illnesses occur with great frequency and are a leading reason that people seek medical help. Depression can cause actual physical symptoms, such as severe headache, digestive disturbance, or weight loss. In addition, relatively minor aches and pains of whatever origin can be greatly accentuated in a depression and may become the entire focus of the patient's thinking.

In the course of the medical evaluation of a depressed patient, the physician may find a condition of relatively little importance and may mention it to the patient. Depressed patients are apt to become totally preoccupied with this finding and may attribute all their misery to it. Many conditions serve this function. Nonfunctioning gallbladder and uterine abnormalities are two typical examples.

Gallbladders have long been depressed people's scapegoat.

In fact, the very term melancholy (melan-black, chole-bile) has its origin in the folk belief that depression was caused by some disorder of the bile. The term "bilious" is defined in the dictionary as "of ill-natured disposition."

Depressed patients with digestive symptoms do indeed deserve a gastrointestinal workup. However, the only abnormality found may at times be a nonfunctioning gallbladder; that is, patients have no gallstones, but their gallbladders do not behave normally on radiographic studies. This may or may not be related to the patients' misery, but desperate patients will grasp at straws. They are relieved to discover a physical abnormality, the correction of which they think will relieve their dejection, loss of appetite, fatigue, and discomfort; and they may be only too happy to undergo surgery. Unfortunately, if the prime problem is really a depressive illness, the symptoms are apt to return with much greater intensity after the immediate post-operative period. The same is true of depressed women who have pelvic discomfort.[1]

A fifty-eight-year-old woman came for psychiatric consultation because of severe depression of more than a year's duration. After the onset of her depression, she had undergone a complete medical evaluation, at which time the gynecologist found a benign tumor of the uterus and said, "That uterus may have to come out some day." She then asked why she could not have the operation promptly, and the doctor explained to her that as long as the growth remained small, she did not need surgery, and she might never require the operation. All he had meant by his remark was that in case the tumor did become larger, it might cause difficulties that would warrant surgery.

The woman said that from that day onward, she thought of nothing else but of having the hysterectomy performed. She

---

[1] S. Merkle, "Psychological Effects of Hysterectomy," *Canadian Psychological Review* 18 (1977): 128–141; R. Martin, N. Roberts, and P. Clayton, "Psychiatric Status After Hysterectomy," *Journal of American Medical Association* 244 (1980): 350–355.

consulted several gynecologists, each time complaining of more severe pelvic pain, until she found a doctor who agreed that she should undergo a hysterectomy. For two weeks after the operation, she felt much better, but then the depressive feelings returned with greater intensity than ever.

This is not at all an uncommon occurrence. Depression is without doubt the most distressing feeling a person can have, as is evidenced by the fact that while few people who suffer from physical pain commit suicide, suicide is unfortunately all too frequent among depressed people. With physical pain, the sufferer often can perceive a tangible cause for the pain, such as a ruptured lumbar disc, a diseased joint, or an obstructed intestine. The awareness of a definitive source of the pain allows patients to speculate that doctors will be able to do something specific to relieve it. In depression, however, all there is is pure misery, and because the patients cannot see what anyone can do to alleviate the distress, they feel that they are doomed to suffer forever. This sense of despair and hopelessness is a major factor in suicide.

If depressive patients have any kind of physical discomfort, they may become so obsessed with the pain that it actually becomes more intense; and when they consult another physician, the pain they describe is so intense that it indeed constitutes legitimate grounds for surgery.

Depression following hysterectomy is not an infrequent occurrence. In some cases, even where there are perfectly valid objective indications for the surgery, the woman may have an emotional reaction, possibly because of her feeling that absence of the uterus takes away from her femininity. In patients who are vulnerable to depression, the physiologic stress of the surgery may precipitate a depression. But in some cases the woman had a pre-existing depression that was masked by the discovery of an abnormality of the uterus, and her depression went untreated while the focus was transferred to the uterus. In these cases, it is typical to find a temporary improvement in the depression once the decision to operate is made, because the patient now looks forward to magical relief from her misery. During the immediate post-operative period, the patient still feels hopeful, attributing her misery to the discomfort that follows surgery. As healing progresses, with the underlying depression remaining untreated, the feelings of dejection begin to return, and those feelings may be expressed in either frank depression or in persistent pelvic pain for which the doctor can find no cause.

Because of the still-lingering stigma attached to mental illness, there is often a collusion between doctor and patient, although neither may be aware of this. The patient does not wish to consider herself as "psycho," and the physician does not want to "accuse" the patient of being "mental." The discovery of a physical abnormality, such as slight elevation of the blood pressure, a mild anemia, or, as mentioned above, a nonfunctioning gallbladder or small uterine fibroid, gives both the doctor and patient a "respectable" alternative.

As an intern, I did an initial history and physical examination of a young woman who had been admitted to the hospital with a diagnosis of "fever of unknown origin." She had no physical discomfort or other symptoms but had discovered that her temperature fluctuated from day-to-day, sometimes reaching 99.8°. I wondered how she had come to take her temperature regularly, because she had no symptoms of illness, thinking that perhaps she was trying to establish the date of ovulation. The patient said that the latter was not the case but that she had been taking her temperature daily for awhile and happened to discover that it was frequently above the accepted normal of 98.6°.

I then noted the physician's orders and found that he had ordered a very extensive workup, including specialized X-ray studies and a host of blood tests. I told him that there was something strange about a young woman who took her temperature daily for no apparent reason, and I suggested that this slight temperature elevation was probably a normal variant. I further suggested that the woman probably has some emotional problem that has made her preoccupied with taking her temperature.

The doctor concurred that the latter might well be the

case. "However," he said, "she might also have a silent cancer some place, and I should give her the *benefit of the doubt.*"

This incident occurred long before I had any psychiatric training, but I recall thinking how strange the doctor's reasoning appeared to me. Granted his desire to perform an extensive physical workup, his term "benefit of the doubt" leaves no alternative to the conclusion that he considered the discovery of a hidden cancer as causative of the temperature elevation to somehow be "beneficial" to the patient, who would otherwise have to be diagnosed as "neurotic" for taking her temperature daily. Confronting the patient with the observation, "Dear, this daily temperature–taking business is a strange thing to do. I'd like you to discuss this with a psychiatrist," would be insulting to her, telling her that she has a psychological problem and is a "mental case." However, if he could walk in and announce, "I have found a malignant tumor," she would be vindicated. She would now have a "real" disease, which, although it might take her life, would not detract from her self-esteem.

Neither the physician nor the patient may be consciously aware of their attitudes; yet the latter can be operative in diverting the doctor from the correct diagnosis, with both doctor and patient becoming involved with the treatment of an incidental and perhaps minor physical problem, while the true disease of depression goes untreated.

Parenthetically, this approach may sometimes be successful, because many depressions are self-limited, and remission eventually occurs even without any psychiatric treatment. But in many cases the depression persists after the physical problem has been resolved, and the doctor or patient may then go on to search for another physical abnormality, or the patient may ultimately be referred for psychiatric help for a depression that may now be more difficult to treat.

The depressed patients whose physical complaints result in abdominal surgery present yet another problem. In the healing process following surgery, scar tissue or adhesions are apt to form, which may interfere with intestinal activity and may cause painful obstruction. If the depression persists and the patients are prone to complain of abdominal pain as a component of their depression, the possibility of intestinal obstruction must be considered each time this symptom occurs, and the patients may end up with repeated hospitalizations and possibly additional surgery.

Doctors have been criticized and accused of performing "unnecessary" surgery. Even if it can be demonstrated that the actual organic pathology did not warrant surgery, the doctor is not necessarily at fault, if we recognize the limitation of psychiatric education and the overwhelming emphasis on physical diseases that prevails in medical education. The green-robed surgeon is the adored hero in the medical school just as on the television screen, and psychiatry is too often the stepchild that is grudgingly accepted despite strong feeling that it does not really "belong." Given this attitude, doctors who are faced with patients complaining bitterly of discomfort and who discover some physical abnormality in patients genuinely believe that they have found the source of the trouble and can relieve the patients' suffering by treating the physical conditions.

A greater awareness of the true role of emotional problems, including their manifestation in physical symptoms and the fact that *people have as much legitimate right to hurt emotionally as they do physically* will permit correct diagnosis and appropriate treatment to take place.

14

What Is Normal?

In 1963, Congress passed the bill that enabled the establishment of a network of Community Mental Health Centers around the country. The need for these appeared obvious. Psychiatrists at that time were relatively scarce, and a person with a pressing emotional problem might have to wait six weeks or longer for an appointment, while the problem required prompt attention. The community mental health center was to resolve this problem by making available skilled mental health professionals working together with psychiatrists. Through these clinics, immediate attention was to be made available.

As the clinics began to function, and there is no question that they have accomplished a great deal of their purpose, they gradually became saturated with patients/clients, and eventually many clinics developed long waiting lists. It is now not unusual to have to wait for a clinic appointment just as long as one had to wait for a private psychiatrist before the clinics came into being.

Some of the patients who seek help at mental health center clinics are people who, prior to the availability of the clinics, not only would have coped with their situations but would not have identified their difficulties as *psychiatric* problems. This does not detract from the fact that the clinics have often been very helpful in providing relief from many unpleasant situations. The point is that people who had not been psychiatric patients became psychiatric patients as the result of the greater availability of psychiatric help. In many instances, what had been a difficult life situation became identified as a psychiatric problem and acquired a medical diagnosis.

Quite often a symptom acquires the status of a symptom only when help is available to relieve it. A "blue day" can become a depression; uneasiness can become anxiety; and laziness can become passive–dependency.

Human life is full of distresses, both physical and emotional. The biblical story of man in paradise teaches that a stress–free blissful life was enjoyed by mankind only briefly, and since the expulsion from the Garden of Eden, man has been subject to all types of unpleasantness.

People adapt to many unpleasant things; they learn to take them in stride. They are particularly apt to do so when they do not see any way of ridding themselves of unpleasantness. These difficulties are perceived as "normal" and are often either ignored or just bemoaned. However, if someone offers a solution or indicates that this unpleasantness can be relieved, the people's tolerance for it drops precipitously. They then feel that suffering unnecessarily is ridiculous and they understandably seek relief. What was previously tolerated as one of the unavoidable drudgeries of life becomes a "symptom."

This state of affairs might have been innocuous except for a few considerations. First of all, a previously "well" person, albeit with problems, has now become a patient or a "sick" person. Secondly, sick people must be "treated," and treatment is not without its pitfalls.

One of the dangers in being treated is that both doctors and patients frequently identify treatment with the prescribing of medication. I was fortunate to have had a teacher in medical school who insisted that medication should never be prescribed unless the doctor has first identified pathology or sickness. He believed, and rightly so, that every biologically active chemical has or can have undesirable side effects and that all administration of medication is a trade-off, such as when the beneficial effects of the medication are sufficiently great to warrant possible undesirable effects. Hence, he said, if you cannot identify anything in the body that needs correction by a chemical, do not introduce any non-nutrient chemical into it.

This was a wise admonition. However, if we consider people to have anxiety and depression rather than being upset as a result of some of the vicissitudes encountered in life, they will become patients with illnesses for which medication may then be justified.

Medications are powerful substances whose effects should not be minimized. Under some conditions they can be extremely helpful and life-saving, under others they can be quite damaging.

The medications most often prescribed for "anxiety" are tranquilizers, many of which can be habituating and addictive. A person who was prescribed 5 mg of Valium three times daily for nervousness may often have to increase the dosage after a period of time because the body had developed a tolerance or immunity to the medication; the original dosage no longer alleviated the distress. Before too long, the body becomes immune to the effect of the increased dosage, so that additional medication is required. I have had patients admitted for addiction to as high as 400 mg of Valium daily, who several years earlier had been prescribed small doses because of "nervousness."

Another group of nerve medications, known as the major tranquilizers, may not be addictive, but some have potentially serious side effects such as uncontrollable muscular movements. These drugs are therefore generally used only in mental illnesses whose severity warrants taking the risk of such side effects. Thus, even in this age of "wonderdrugs" there are really no completely safe tranquilizers. Yet, the availablity of medications that can relieve the discomforts of tension has led to the latter's often being considered an abnormal symptom that justifies being treated rather than a reaction to normal stress.

Psychotherapy for relief of unpleasant feelings, while not carrying with it the risk of chemical side effects or addiction, is not completely free of risk. Some types of psychotherapy can produce more trouble than they set out to relieve.

In the mid-twentieth century, the theories of Sigmund Freud gained immense popularity. Freud was unquestionably a psychological genius whose systematic investigation of the unconscious mind is without equal in the history of psychology. Many of his findings were new and stimulating and held out hope that they would lead to the resolution of many mental conditions. Freud's followers and successors modified his theories or took off on axes of their own, with the resultant emergence of numerous schools of dynamic psychiatry. Although differing in many ways, these schools generally share the belief that the understanding and uncovering of the source of a mental symptom can result in its elimination.

The most profound emotional effects that are considered in dynamic psychiatry are those stemming from the interactions with those people closest to us. Since much of personality formation occurs in the early years of life, the impact of parents on one's psychological makeup is of course most significant. Relationships with siblings are also of extreme importance. Later on in life interactions with spouses and children are of major importance.

The assumption in dynamic psychiatry that emotional disorders are the consequence of interpersonal trauma and deprivation in childhood generally leads to investigation of these events in therapy. While the theory is sound and probably correct, the therapeutic applications are often fraught with hazard. What happens all too often is that significant people in patients' lives begin to be perceived as villains and as the cause of their misery. Children are turned against parents and vice versa, and spouses and siblings are set against one another.

The fallacy is not in the theory. I like to think of the investigation of dynamics as analogous to the study of anatomy, which is accomplished by dissection of a body. Familiarity with the positions and relationships of various anatomical organs, which medical students acquire by meticulous dissection of a human body, enables them later as physicians to interpret symptoms presented by patients in terms of which organs may be involved. Upon concluding which organ is affected, physicians can further direct their tests and treatment. However, it is obviously not necessary that they perform dissections on every patient that they see. Similarly, a thorough understanding of the workings of the psychological entity should serve as a basis for therapists to understand how some symptom or personality trait developed. It is not often essential to perform a meticulous dissection in which the patient is an active participant and which can unfortunately lead to distortions by both the patient and the therapist.

The entire area of causality of emotional problems is therapeutically hazardous. Even if the cause of a problem can be identified with absolute certainty, it does not necessarily follow that its discovery will contribute significantly to alleviation of the patient's ills. Think of a house on fire, where it is known that a lit cigarette ignited the flame. Responsible firefighters put out the fire instead of searching for the cigarette while the house goes up in smoke.

Searching for the cause of a problem may have yet another danger. In many instances, overcoming a neurotic symptom or a dysfunctional trait may require a great deal of effort on the part of the patient. Behavior patterns, no matter how unhealthy, are not easily reversed, as evidenced by the difficulty often encountered by people who wish to stop smoking. People have a natural resistance to change and a tendency to circumvent change in any possible way.

The search for the cause of a psychological symptom often leads to "scapegoating," when the patients believe they have found the source of their misery and rather than undergo the discomfort necessary to overcome the problem, are satisfied with the status quo as long as they have someone to blame. Take, for example, the lazy or "passive–dependent" person who is getting nowhere in life and who is helped in therapy to discover that his mother was a very needy, insecure person who was deprived of affection by a cold, uncaring husband. He learns that she therefore overprotected her child to the point of infantilizing him and not preparing him adequately for the assertiveness and competitiveness necessary to make one's way in the world. Changing his behavior would require such sacrifices as getting out of bed early in the morning, going out to look for work, accepting the discomfort of rejection, accepting the responsibility of a job and the authority of superiors, competing with others, and always being at risk of losing what he has attained. These are all distinctly unpleasant, and it is unquestionably much easier to consider oneself an innocent victim of a set of parents who were derelict in child-rearing. One can then wallow in perhaps justifiable wrath, angry at parents, grandparents, older siblings, and God. Insights acquired in therapy may thus be completely true while also totally useless.

Resistance to change should not be underestimated. Therapists may have every good intention in imparting etiologic insights, but patients may use these in their own way to perpetuate the pathology rather than the way the therapists hope they would use them.

The foregoing remarks should not be taken as a criticism of insight-oriented psychotherapy. In many situations this is an effective modality in skilled hands. The criticism is intended primarily for those therapists who have not been adequately trained in the application of depth psychotherapy and for the popular practice of "psyching out" oneself or one's family members.

Many highly skilled therapists know what to do with dynamics and use the etiologic insights they derive from the patients' histories to enable *them* to relate to the patients in a manner that facilitates the changes the patients must make in their behaviors. Perhaps a good general rule would be: etiologic insights are for the therapist, not necessarily for the patient. The patients' insights should be into what it is that they are doing, of which they may be unaware. The patients should be helped to put out the fire rather than look for the match.

Not all therapists observe this rule, and if people bring an emotional problem to one of these, they risk becoming estranged from parents, siblings, and spouse, all of whom may love and care for the patients in the only way they know. The separation resulting from such estrangement almost always aggravates the patients' miseries or leads them into ill-advised escapist maneuvers such as unsound marriage or divorce. Thus, well-intended psychotherapy, just as well-intended medication, is not without risk.

In some situations the psychotherapy required is along the lines of counseling and direction, or helping people fully use or develop effective coping skills. This is not equivalent to the advice offered by a well-meaning friend, and this type of psychotherapy can require as great an expertise as that of the more classical variety. A subtle but significant distinction is that the problem is then perceived as one of life's stresses, and the people who seek help with this are not classified as being mentally ill. Another derivative of this approach is that the idea of coping with stress implies effort on the part of the patient and is understood to entail some difficult adjustments, whereas the illness paradigm may set up unrealistic expectations in the patient that the doctor as the purveyor of modern medicine has the magic potion or the therapeutic touch that will instantaneously relieve the discomfort.

Far beyond being a matter of semantics, the determination of whether a given behavior is normal or abnormal has great therapeutic implications. It therefore behooves us to try to refine our conceptualization of normality and abnormality and to further fine-tune the latter as to what type of abnormality exists, if we are to maximize available help and eliminate therapeutic misadventures.

15

Therapy
of Distress

Evelyn is a forty-four-year-old woman who was out bowling with friends one evening when she was called to the phone. She sensed that something terrible must have happened, because she had never been traced down this way before. The call was from a neighbor, who had just been notified by the hospital that Evelyn's husband had been brought to the emergency room, having collapsed at the office with an apparent heart attack. Evelyn had often pleaded with her husband not to go back to the office at night, but she could not stop Harold.

It was a while before they let Evelyn into the coronary care unit. Harold was sedated but was able to smile to her and say a few words. The chest pain had occurred with sudden intensity, although he admitted that he had experienced mild episodes of chest pressure in the few preceding weeks, which he had chosen to ignore.

Harold was connected by wire to several machines, and Evelyn was frightened by the wavy green streaks that made their way across the television screen and by the blinking of red lights that seemed to indicate to her that something was about to stop. She knew that these machines were monitoring her husband's heartbeat, and she was terrified by the thought that his heart might stop.

The following day Harold's doctor was cautious in reassuring Evelyn. Harold's heart attack was one of the severest he had seen, and all the tests pointed to extensive heart muscle damage. The first forty-eight hours were the most crucial, he said, but not until a full ten days had passed would Harold be considered out of danger.

Evelyn returned to an empty house. Their two children were both away at school, and she had informed them of their father's condition. Seeing Arthur through law school and Nora through college was costly. Would Harold's illness interfere with the children's education and careers? She tried to fight off the terrible thought, but what if Harold did not survive the danger period? How would she continue to keep the children in school? Had Harold provided for this? She had never talked to Harold about his insurance. Oh, God! How could she think such selfish thoughts while Harold was lying there fighting for his life?

Evelyn turned on the light in the living room. The room was beautifully furnished; in fact, it was just one year to the day that they had moved into their new home. This had been a major financial undertaking, and perhaps she should not have allowed Harold to extend himself. Of course, she had wanted the house, and Harold knew she had been dissatisfied with where they had been living. Three years earlier, her sister Caroline had bought a sumptuous new home, and Evelyn had always felt that she could not catch up with Caroline. But then Caroline's husband did not have to go back to the office to work nights. He could leave for several days vacation anytime he wished. Evelyn was jealous of Caroline, and at times she hated Caroline for being better off than she.

What would happen to the home if Harold did not recover? She did not know the exact figures, because Harold had never familiarized her with any of their financial details. "Don't you worry," he would say. "Making the money is my job. Spending it is yours." Evelyn knew that Harold would do anything to keep her happy. But had she really needed the house for happiness?

During the first three days in the hospital, Harold's condition was stable, but on the fourth day, the doctor's ominous

warning came to pass. Harold's heart had stopped twice, but
both times he was successfully resuscitated. Evelyn did not
leave the hospital all that day, and only toward midnight, when
the nurse told her that Harold was resting comfortably, did she
return home for sleep.

At 3:00 A.M., the phone rang, and Evelyn knew that this
could not be good. She was to come to the hospital immediately.
They had not said so over the phone, but as Evelyn got dressed,
she knew that the worst had happened.

The children stayed with her for two days after the funeral,
but then had to return to school. Eugene, Evelyn's older brother,
offered to return in a week to help straighten out all the fiscal
intricacies. There were so many papers, none of which Evelyn
had seen before. Loans, banks, correspondence with attorneys,
brokerage transactions, insurance policies—they all seemed so
confusing. Evelyn had never even reconciled the check book
before. Harold had always taken care of everything.

A will? Harold did not appear to have made one. His at-
torney said that Harold had said something about going into
the office to draw up a will but had never actually done so.

"How could he do this to me?" Evelyn thought. "Why
hadn't he familiarized me with all that we owed and owned?
Why didn't he leave a will?" Evelyn forced herself to stop
thinking this way because she felt herself becoming angry at
Harold, and it wasn't right to be angry at someone for whom
one was grieving.

Two weeks after Harold's death, Eugene came, and he was
indeed a great help. He noticed that Evelyn appeared very drawn
and haggard. Evelyn confided that she had not been sleeping
well at all and had not been eating much. She had difficulty
cooking for one person, she said. Eugene called the doctor, who
prescribed some medication for sleep and a tranquilizer three
times daily to "take the edge off."

The children called almost every night, and their calls were
a welcome respite, but Evelyn did not bother them with the

myriad troubles of the day. They were in school and did not
need their heads burdened by her problems. When Eugene
returned five weeks later to help tie up some loose ends, he
noted that Evelyn had lost weight and appeared depressed. With
the help of Evelyn's doctor, Eugene was able to arrange an
appointment with a psychiatrist.

About a year later Evelyn was admitted to the hospital,
having taken an overdose of sleeping pills. During her evaluation,
doctors learned that Evelyn had been taking sleeping pills and
tranquilizers regularly since Harold's death. Her family physician
had continued to prescribe refills at Evelyn's request and probably had not noted that the usage of the pills had increased. In
recent months, Evelyn was taking three pills each night to
sleep. The doctor had also refilled her tranquilizer prescription
frequently.

Evelyn's psychiatrist had prescribed antidepressant medication and another type of tranquilizer. Evelyn had not told the
psychiatrist about the medication her family physician had given
her because she felt she just might need "something extra." She
thus was taking sedative and tranquilizing drugs in addictive
fashion.

According to Evelyn's account, much of the time she spent
in the psychiatrist's office had been devoted to ventilating her
feelings of envy and hostility toward her sister Caroline and to
working through her anger toward Harold for leaving her so
totally unprepared, although not unprovided for. Undoubtedly,
what the psychiatrist was trying to do was to help Evelyn with
the grief process, which was "derailed," as it were, by her hostile
feelings. Unfortunately, little or nothing could have been accomplished psychotherapeutically with a brain that was under
constant sedation.

A review of Evelyn's case points out a glaring error. Evelyn
was initially given various kinds of psychotropic medication
although there was no indication that she was sick.

Evelyn had indeed been sleepless, agitated, and even depressed. But consider the circumstances: Her husband had died suddenly. Her children were away from home, and she was totally alone. Having been completely unfamiliar with financial management, she was suddenly overwhelmed with many fiscal problems that were very confusing to her. She was indeed intensely upset and worried by all of this. Evelyn was in considerable distress, but was there anything abnormal about the way she felt? Was it not perfectly normal and understandable for someone in her circumstances to feel and react the way she did? Is grief not a normal reaction? Is worry about not knowing how to manage finances not normal? What indication is there that Evelyn was "sick?" And if she was not sick, why was she given medication? The right medication can be very effective when they address a disease, but no medication can be of benefit when no illness exists.

Evelyn's initial symptoms were of grief rather than depression. The first physician tried to help, but apparently his understanding of help was to prescribe medication that would reduce the distress. Evelyn's feelings, although very painful, were nevertheless healthy. The help she needed at this time was to go through the grief process, get the grief worked on, and then be in a position to readjust to life. The medication she was given unfortunately stifled the grief process, so that it progressed into a clinical depression.

Consulting the psychiatrist was indeed a wise move, but it, too, miscarried. At this point, Evelyn had two problems. First, she had the reality problem of losing her husband and all the adjustments consequent to this loss, including the many details for whose management she had been unprepared. Second, she had depressive illness that had been precipitated by the loss and by the interruption of the grieving process. This was probably not adequately grasped by the significant people in Evelyn's environment. They understood that she was "sick," and thus felt assured that the doctor would get her "well." They probably did not realize that a part of Evelyn's distress consisted also of healthy pain, of the suffering one undergoes upon the loss of someone close. Nor did they realize that for this healthy aspect of Evelyn's distress, they themselves could provide significant help of a kind that was beyond the realm of the psychiatrist; namely, the closeness and the sharing of the grief, the value of which is reflected in the adage, "Joy that is shared is doubled; grief that is shared is halved."

Modern medicine has good reason to be proud. Grave illnesses that were at one time fatal have been conquered, and significant progress is being made in many other areas. Transplant surgery that just a short while ago was science–fiction material is now a reality. Wonder drugs exist whose effects border on the miraculous.

The high esteem in which medicine is held has an unfortunate drawback: people often expect more from doctors than they can provide. Particularly, doctors are frequently expected to solve *all* problems, whether or not they are related to illness. This is a serious fallacy. Doctors are able to provide treatment for illness; reality adjustments generally require something other than a doctor's ministrations.

Evelyn had a good family. They undoubtedly would have provided more support had they been aware that she needed it. Their error was that they relied on the psychiatrist to do *everything*—their share as well as his own job. They did not appreciate that her seeing the psychiatrist once a week did not provide all the outlet she required.

This was further complicated by another cultural error. People have a natural tendency to avoid pain and distress, as evidenced by the reflex pulling away of one's hand from a hot stove. Our culture reinforces this with a media bombardment of numerous nostrums to relieve various sorts of distress. The concept of "healthy" distress has become alien to our culture.

All members of a family in which there has been a tragic

death experience the distress of sorrow. In instances such as
Evelyn's, the family members sometimes do talk to each other
about their husband, father, and brother. Each has experienced
the loss in his own way. They cry together, and even in their
mourning, can manage to smile together when memories of
pleasant events are recalled.

Too often, however, this mourning is not maximized.
Sometimes this is because of the various family members being
dispersed and not being in close contact. Sometimes it is because of the tendency to change the subject when the conversation leads to pain.

Back in my days as a rabbi, I was called to officiate at
funeral services for a little child of three. The child had escaped
her mother's usual watchful eye and had run off to play. As
soon as the mother noted her absence, she began looking for
her. The child was subsequently found drowned in a nearby
pool.

The grief of the parents and the extended family was
intense. When I visited the home, I noted that everyone left
the room, leaving only the mother and myself. The mother
would then begin to recount the events and, while crying pro-
fusely, would relate how she had only looked away momentarily
and how it had never occurred to her to immediately check the
pool. She would talk of how beautiful the child was, how bright
she was, and how everyone had loved her. This pattern recurred
every time I visited the home. Upon my entry, all others would
exit, and the mother would unburden herself.

I subsequently learned from some of the family members
that every time the mother began to talk about the tragedy, they
would divert her to some other subject. They said that they
could not bear the pain that this aroused in them nor could
they watch her cry and grieve. It was only when I came and
they all left that she had the opportunity to ventilate.

In Evelyn's case, the combination of her children being

away at school and the reluctance of the family to talk about Harold deprived her of sufficient outlets for her expression of grief. Her pastor might have been very helpful, but because the family assumed that Evelyn was "only sick," and that she was being adequately treated for her illness, they did not involve the pastor. An unrealistic burden was placed upon the psychiatrist, whose best ministrations could not fulfill Evelyn's healthy needs as well as treat the illness aspects of her depression.

The success of self-help groups such as Alcoholics Anonymous may be largely because of the help provided in coping with reality problems. Traditional insight–oriented psychiatric treatment of the alcoholic is generally less effective than Alcoholics Anonymous, and this is undoubtedly because the majority of alcoholics do not suffer from pathological anxiety but rather from an inability to cope with *normal* anxiety. They need help in coping with normality, and if they seek psychiatric or psychologic help, the course may follow the path of searching for the sources of pathological anxiety that may be nonexistent. Recovered alcoholics know little about pathology but have expertise in how to adjust to sundry reality difficulties, an expertise that even an expert psychotherapist, unless trained in the treatment of alcoholism, does not necessarily have.

Loss of job, foreclosure on a home, rejection by a spouse, having a child with serious birth defects or a parent who becomes senile, failure of one's business—these are some of the traumata that may befall a person, and these result in great distress. While such distress is difficult to tolerate, it is on the whole quite normal. In fact, *not to be distressed* under such circumstances would be unusual. Normal distress, no matter how difficult, should not be confused with emotional illness. The sufferer may need any and every kind of support, both moral and material, that the family and community can provide, and psychotherapy may be beneficial in correcting overreactions or other inappropriate responses; but unless an actual emotional illness becomes

superimposed on the normal distress reaction, "treatment" and
medication are not appropriate. Many treatment failures in psychiatry may be caused by the fact that the patient was not sick
to begin with.[1]

[1]"Help the Patient through Major Loss," *Patient Care*, M. Alderman,
editor, Vol. 17 (February 1983) 57–64.

16

There Is Nothing Wrong with You

It was about 3:00 A.M. when the ambulance pulled up in the emergency room entrance. The two paramedics gently lifted the stretcher, which bore a female patient with an oxygen mask in place over her nose and mouth.

The nurse took the information from the paramedics. The patient's blood pressure was normal and stable. The heart rate was somewhat rapid but the rhythm was regular. They had received the call at 2:15 A.M. and were at the scene by 2:25 A.M. The patient had complained of chest pain and shortness of breath.

With the help of the paramedics, Beatrice was transferred from the stretcher to a bed in the emergency room. The nurse made her comfortable, and, as she attached the wires of the heart monitor, she assured Beatrice that there did not appear to be any reason for alarm and that she should try to relax. She took Beatrice's blood pressure and made a notation on the chart.

Shortly thereafter a young physician entered the room. He glanced up at the monitor, then asked Beatrice, "What seems to be the trouble?"

"Pain right across here," Beatrice said, drawing her hand across her midchest from side-to-side. "Not so much pain as pressure, like being caught in a vise. It cuts off my breathing. I can't seem to get any air."

"Ever have anything like this before?" the doctor asked.

"No," Beatrice said. "It just came over me while I was lying in bed."

"Did you ever notice any chest pain or shortness of breath when you climbed stairs or exerted yourself?" the doctor asked.

Beatrice shook her head. "No. I live on the third floor and always walk up two flights of stairs without any problem."

The doctor proceeded to inquire about Beatrice's medical history. She was fifty-eight and except for common colds had never been sick before. Her only hospitalization had been for childbirth. The doctor asked about illnesses in her family and about the causes of her parents' deaths. He then proceeded to listen to Beatrice's heart and lungs and completed a fairly thorough physical examination.

A young man clad in white came in and took several tubes of blood. He was followed by a nurse who started an intravenous administration of glucose. The doctor said something to the nurse and then addressed Beatrice. "You're going to get an injection to help you relax. After a bit we'll have a chest X-ray taken. Right now everything looks okay, though. I see no reason for you to worry."

Outside Beatrice's room the doctor said to the nurse, "All the symptoms point to an infarct, but the EKG looks good.[1] Rather unlikely to have an infarct without any previous angina on exertion, but it can happen. She's not diabetic, hypertensive, overweight, and doesn't smoke, but it still could be. Also have to think of a pulmonary embolism.[2] Can't find any source for it, but we should get a lung scan. Have her admitted to coronary care."

Beatrice rested her head on the pillow. She hoped that the doctor was right. The pressure on her chest was still there, and although she could feel the jets of oxygen in her nostrils, she still felt that she could not get enough air. The nurse came in

[1]A heart attack.
[2]A blood clot in the lung.

bearing a syringe. "Over on your side a bit," she said. "Just a little pin prick."

A few minutes later Beatrice felt the pressure easing, her breathing becoming much less labored, and she became drowsy, soon drifting into a deep sleep.

Beatrice awoke in the coronary care unit. She was in a little cubicle, and she was attached by wires to several machines. Her oxygen catheter was in place and the intravenous fluid was dripping slowly.

A nurse came to her bedside. "Good to see you're up," she said. "Everything looks fine. Your daughter is out in the waiting room and we were waiting to let her in until you awoke. We'll call her in now."

Beatrice was glad to see Cathy, who kissed her gently on the forehead. "Everything is going to be okay, Mother," Cathy said. "I talked to the doctor and he said that everything is checking out well." Cathy went on to tell Beatrice that the children were all fine and that she had gotten them off to school. She had called off work that day. "I called Steve," she said. "He'll be in after work." Steve was Cathy's fiancé.

Beatrice became aware of the pain in her chest, although it was not as severe as it had been. She patted Cathy's hand. "I'll be all right," she said.

The next two days were spent answering questions posed by several doctors. The same thing over and over again. When had she first noticed the pain, and what was its character? Did it stay in one place or did it radiate to her arm or shoulder? Had she ever had pain on exertion? Had she eaten a heavy meal that night? What had her parents died of? Beatrice had said to Cathy, "Why do they all ask the same questions over and over? Can't they just read what the doctor wrote?"

Cathy suggested, "They probably can't read the doctor's handwriting." They both laughed.

There were repeated blood tests and a few trips to the X-ray. The intravenous fluid was discontinued, and Beatrice was allowed to walk down the hall and sit in the waiting room with Cathy.

On the third day Beatrice and Cathy were talking when one of the young doctors came in and said, "We have good news for you, Mrs. Young. You may go home today. There's nothing wrong with you."

Cathy threw her arms around her mother. "See, mom, I told you everything would be all right," she said. Tears welled up in Beatrice's eyes. "Why are you crying, Mother?" Cathy asked. "You heard what the doctor said. You're all right. There is nothing wrong with you."

"It's just that I'm so happy that everything's okay," Beatrice said. "I had been so worried." Beatrice turned to the doctor. "What about the pain?" she asked.

"Nothing to worry about," the doctor said. "Your heart is fine and your lungs are clear. Nothing wrong with you."

The next morning Beatrice arose at the usual early hour. Cathy and the children were still asleep. She set about preparing their breakfast as usual, then she gathered the laundry that had accumulated during her three-day absence and prepared it for washing.

Beatrice wondered what life would be like after Steve and Cathy married. The house would be empty. No clothes to prepare, very little laundry to do, no one to pick up after, and she really didn't know how to cook for one person or whether it was worth the bother.

These were the same thoughts that had gone through Beatrice's mind when she went to bed that night that she became ill. That evening Cathy had told her that she and Steve were going to get married. Steve had been offered a promotion in his firm, but this would mean that he would be moving to another city. Beatrice was very happy for Cathy, who had been divorced for five years and who certainly deserved the happiness and security of marriage for herself and her three children.

Beatrice had been unable to fall asleep that night. The

thoughts of the approaching loneliness were frightening. What would motivate her to get out of bed in the morning? With Cathy and the children hundreds of miles away, what reason would there be for her going through the motions of living? Not that Beatrice ever thought of taking her own life, but life suddenly was losing all interest. Beatrice chided herself for thinking this way. How could she be so selfish, feeling sorry for herself, when she should be exulted over Cathy's good fortune?

Beatrice had tossed and turned, unable to fall asleep. It was then that she noticed the first twinge of pain, which then just became progressively worse and seemed to cut off her breathing.

Human beings are very complicated organisms. Physiologists describe automatic protective responses and intricate defensive mechanisms that are operative within people that are totally beyond their awareness and completely beyond their volitional control.

Psychologists assure us that the physiologic responses are more than paralleled by psychological defenses and maneuvers, which are also independent of our volition and proceed beyond our awareness.

Beatrice was clearly in considerable turmoil on that night when her chest pain occurred. Not only had she become aware of a major change that would be forthcoming in her life, not only had she become most apprehensive about what meaning life would hold for her after her children left, but she also struggled with further conflict and guilt for even thinking about herself and for not being euphoric about her daughter's happiness. Had Beatrice stubbed her toe, she would have screamed "ouch!" without any self-reproach about feeling pain. But this was different. Although Beatrice was hurting badly, she did not have the luxury of permitting herself to feel the pain.

This internal conflict raged within her at about 1:00 A.M. Perhaps had Beatrice been able to unburden herself to someone, her distress might have been alleviated somewhat. If someone could also have encouraged her unburdening and reassured her that it was all right to feel the way she did, that joy and resentment could coexist and be experienced by one and the same individual, and that she was not a bad person for feeling the way she did, Beatrice would have been greatly relieved.

But all of this occurred at 1:00 A.M. To whom could she talk at 1:00 A.M.? The only sources of help available at 1:00 A.M. are hospital emergency staff, and one does not go there to talk about difficult life situations and stresses.

The human unconscious is unbelievably shrewd and efficient. In fact, all the vital functions of the body that are all ultimately under control of the brain are regulated by the unconscious. The conscious mind is simply not to be trusted with the regulation of breathing, heart rate, blood presure, and metabolism. It is only the much wiser unconscious that can be trusted with the very essentials of life.

Beatrice's unconscious mind performed a kind of conversion maneuver that her conscious mind was not clever enough to do, and this was to convert the emotional stress to something that could be relevant and acceptable to the only source of help available at 1:00 A.M. The emotional stress was thus converted into chest pain and shortness of breath, and these were perfectly legitimate complaints to bring to the attention of the paramedics and the hospital emergency personnel.

Beatrice was not malingering, not putting on an act, and not imagining her symptoms. She was hurting, physically hurting. She was short of air, really gasping for breath. The symptoms were no less severe than those caused by blockage of a blood vessel to the heart or a clot lodging in the lung.

The diagnostic work-up of the hospital was thorough and appropriate. However, the doctor's conclusion was completely erroneous. The negative electrocardiogram, blood test, and lung scan warranted the conclusion: "We cannot find any disease process in your heart and lungs." There was no justification for the conclusion "there is nothing wrong with you." If nothing had been wrong with Beatrice, she would not have felt the pain or have been short of breath.

Once it became apparent that she had no chest disease, doctors should have considered that Beatrice's pain might have been a stress reaction. This is by no means making a diagnosis by exclusion but rather is investigating whether something in Beatrice's life could have produced her symptoms. If such factors were uncovered, Beatrice could then have been referred to an appropriate source of help.

The doctor reached a faulty conclusion because of the kind of mentality prevalent in many medical schools and among many physicians, which considers the human being to be a conglomerate of organs, much like a complicated piece of machinery. The contention that is sometimes made that physicians can be replaced by sophisticated computers would be justified if this were indeed the case.

But a person is more than a machine. Even if computer scientists can develop a machine that "thinks," they will never develop one that feels. Beatrice was "feeling," and all the laboratory studies could not detect her feelings.

However, the doctor, like the patient, is a person. He, too, should feel, unless, of course, his medical training strips him of emotion and converts him into a computer.

This is what happened to Beatrice. All the data available—the history, physical examination, X-rays, ECG's, and blood tests—were fed into the doctor–computer, and he produced a computerized print out: "There is nothing wrong with you."

Pain does not necessarily mean something is wrong with an organ. Pain means that the *person* is hurting. The doctor missed the diagnosis. Several thousands of dollars were spent on Beatrice's three-day hospitalization, but Beatrice was not helped in the way she should have been.

17

The Pain Problem

The confusion of physical versus emotional is often seen in the problem of the management of chronic pain. Patients with persistent complaints of pain are often referred to psychiatrists because someone has determined that the pain is "all in the head," while others undergo procedure after procedure and treatment after treatment for pain for which no physical origin can be found.

Pain is the most common symptom bringing a person to the physician. Pain is generally the body's way of alerting the person that something is wrong. Pain is also a challenge to physicians, for they are taught in medical school that doctors can "cure sometimes, relieve always." Failure to relieve pain is often viewed by physicians as a fundamental failure in their mission and a dereliction of duty.

Pain may be divided into two types: acute pain and chronic pain. It is regrettable that we do not have two totally different terms for these two types of symptoms, because they are very different. Chronic pain differs from acute pain qualitatively, but because the same term "pain" is used for both, they are too often identified with each other, and this may result in the mismanagement of the problem.

Acute pain is of relatively brief duration. It is often related to tissue damage: an injury or disease that is clearly evident. It generally responds well to medication, and, as the injury or disease heals, the pain disappears. The pain generally does not result in disruption of one's life style or relationships. Its mechanism is fairly well elucidated. The medical student learns about nerve fibers that convey pain sensations from external and internal stimuli to the brain, and these teachings appear to be quite sound. Thus the origin, mechanism, and treatment of acute pain are simple.

Precisely the reverse can be said of chronic pain, pain that persists after the injured body tissues have healed and everything appears to be in order. It is difficult if not impossible to determine where the pain comes from, how it is transmitted to the brain, and what to do for it. Neurosurgeons who have tried to relieve chronic pain by cutting the known nerve pathways that carry acute pain sensations generally throw up their hands in surrender. "We can cut every pain tract known to mankind, and the pain still persists." Treatment of chronic pain by means of potent narcotics or narcotic-like drugs often results in the tragedy of addiction, which is further aggravated by the fact that although the patient's life may be ruined by addiction, the pain stubbornly persists in spite of high dosage of drugs.

Typical of chronic pain are low-back pain, pain following injuries or surgery if persistent, and headaches, as well as the pain of the "phantom limb"—the pain felt in the arm or leg that has been amputated.

In many of these cases, examination after examination by all methods known to medicine fail to reveal the source of the pain. Faced by a complaint for which he can find no origin, the doctor may say to the patient, "The pain is all in your head. You should see a psychiatrist." The patient, who feels intense pain in his back or limb, resents what he understands as an implication that he is either malingering or that he is crazy. Unfortunately, the doctor who diagnoses the patient as having a psychogenic pain sometimes has the same concept as the patient and may indeed feel that the patient is either faking or imagining the pain. Nothing can cause greater resentment or alienation than being told that the terrible distress one feels is a "put-on."

Psychogenic pain does indeed exist, but this does not mean that the patients are mentally ill or faking, nor does it mean that they need to undergo psychiatric treatment.

Our bodies often react in ways over which we generally have little or no control. Enter into a brightly illuminated room and your pupils will contract, or go into a darkened room and they will dilate, and there is nothing you can do to prevent this reaction. Visit the place where you were involved in a near–fatal accident, and you may find your heart palpitating, your head spinning, and that you are breaking out in a cold sweat; nothing you can do about this. You are served a tasty dish similar to one that you had been eating when you witnessed a horrible accident, and you find yourself becoming nauseated; you can do nothing about this. The body has its own memory bank and ways of responding, and the latter can often be altered only by persistent and laborious retraining.

Things associated with painful sensations can program the body to produce pain. For example, take the patient who receives narcotic medication for pain. The relief of pain is itself a pleasant experience, but in addition the medication may produce other desirable sensations: euphoria, relief of anxiety and tension, or removal of depressive sensations. The human body is a quick learner and after several doses discovers that if it feels pain, it soon gets a pleasant sensation when it is given a certain medication. The body may then, on its own, *produce real pain*, to get what it wants. This pain can be as severe and as real as the pain of a fracture or other injury. It is not "imaginary" or "put-on."

People who experience pain may find that rest relieves the pain, and their bodies may then produce pain to get the rest they would not otherwise get. Their families may react to their pain with empathy or greater attention and care, and their bodies may produce pain to elicit these responses from the environment.

Physicians who feel frustrated because patients continue to complain in spite of their best treatment efforts may say, "They are complaining of pain because they want drugs, or because they don't want to go to work or do anything around the house, or because they want attention." This is an accusation that the patients are manipulating and makes the patients angry at the doctors, and everyone in the patients' environments angry at the patients. It is not understood that often the patients cannot tell their bodies what to do or what and how to feel.

Some people may indeed manipulate or try to exploit their illness or injury, but others who have no intention of being deceptive nevertheless have complaints of pain which *appear to be* exploitive or manipulative.

Sometimes depressive illnesses manifest themselves primarily in painful symptoms, and in these instances appropriate psychiatric treatment of the depression is very helpful. Often the chronic pain and its disabling effects produce depressive symptoms; here, too, psychiatric treatment of the depression can be helpful. But in many cases the psychiatrist is stymied. Here the patients are really at a loss, because no one seems to be able to help them. Not only do they suffer with severe pain, but everyone is fed up with them and is accusing them of malingering. In their desperation they may begin making the rounds of doctors, and too often will find someone who will either try to operate in the hope of finding something treatable by surgery or who will prescribe potent pain-killing medications that may lead to addiction, or both.

Of course, the most effectual approach to chronic pain problems is prevention. At the first indication that the pain is persisting longer than warranted by the degree of tissue damage, the doctor should curtail the prescription of potent pain-killing drugs and should have a conference with the patient and immediate family members. The limitation of effective medical treatment for chronic pain should be pointed out frankly and empathetically. If at all possible, consultation with an expert on pain management should be obtained, as well as a psychiatric evaluation for the possibility of a depressive illness. The physician should understand and also convey to the patient that the pain may be very real although not produced by actual tissue damage and that the patient is not being considered a malingerer or a neurotic.

At this point in the development of medicine, an insufficient number of comprehensive pain treatment centers are available. The need for more of such treatment programs is great and will likely continue to increase as medical science progresses in prolonging lives of people with serious illnesses and injuries.

A comprehensive pain center comprises a variety of specialists whose combined knowledge can enable a better understanding of patients and their pain problems and provide the various treatment modalities to bring about maximum relief and optimal function. A well-coordinated program may avoid the pitfalls of futile surgical procedures, drug addiction, or the labeling of the patient as a malingerer. The solution to chronic pain is not simple, but the alternatives of being crippled by pain, ruined by addiction, or both, are unacceptable.

18

Some Suggestions

Much is said about considering the patient as a "whole," but in practical terms, this is not adequately implemented.

The broadening scope of human behavior is giving rise to ever-expanding bodies of knowledge in medicine, psychology, and social studies. No one person can master the enormity of all relevant disciplines. The ideal answer is the multi- and interdisciplinary team method, and efforts should be made to approach this ideal as closely as possible.

Although it is unrealistic for any single discipline to cover all the various fields, we must get to know what the others are doing, what they are looking for, how these aspects impinge on what we are doing, and how we can make use of each other's expertise to maximize services to the patient.

In those mental health centers where the multidisciplinary approach is practical, case seminars provide an excellent foundation not only for amalgamating the various aspects of a patient's problems but also for familiarizing each provider with the insights and services that others provide. Physicians are exposed to insights into patients' milieus provided by social workers. They can see how the patients impact and are impacted upon by their families, and how the symptoms, rather than being in the abdomen or neck, may be symptoms of the family unit. Psychologists shed light on the defensive or adaptive character of the patients' illnesses. Psychiatrists discuss the psychological and/or pathologic physical findings in the patients' work-ups, and the role of medications in the patients' treatments. Everyone can see how each facet is an interdependent part of the whole. A case discussion such as this not only serves to provide a unified and comprehensive treatment for the patient under discussion but also alerts therapists to important aspects of symptomatology and therapy that they can apply in the management of other patients.

In some psychiatric centers, courses are available for non-psychiatric physicians to provide greater familiarity with psychosomatic concepts and with how a symptom or malfunction of an organ or system may be the expression of an emotional stress or conflict. As the cases that have been cited indicate, the reverse is also true. A high index of suspicion that a given problem may have physiologic substrata can set the therapist and patient in the right direction, and courses in "somatopsychic" diseases can provide the awareness for both psychiatrists and nonmedical mental health professionals.

Practitioners who are not involved in teaching centers should try to overcome the professional isolation that a busy practice can foster. Continuing professional education should cover significant contributions of other fields. As the cases cited in this book indicate, psychiatrists, psychologists, and other mental health practitioners should have seminars in which the role of physiological disorders affecting human behavior is discussed.

Many psychologists and other mental health practitioners require that any patient who presents symptoms of depression and anxiety undergo a thorough medical evaluation. This is a wise practice. It is regrettable that in some mental health centers, funding for medical evaluation is not always available for the patient who does not have any medical coverage.

For the person who seeks medical help of any type, it would be wise to have a "primary–care physician," a doctor who can coordinate all one's health concerns.

Too often, people seek out specialists for treatment of a particular problem on their own. A given patient may see an allergist for her asthma, a rheumatologist for her arthritis, a psychiatrist for her depression, a gynecologist for her pelvic symptoms, and an ophthalmologist for her visual problem but yet not have one physician who considers the person *as a whole*. A person may have nine or ten specialists, some of whom may not be aware of all the patient's health problems or what another physician may be prescribing. Sometimes the pharmacist who fills the patient's prescription detects an incompatibility or duplication; for example, if the patient is receiving medication from different physicians that either should not be taken together or have the same activity, in which latter case the patient may actually be overdosing.

While there is no proven method to avoid all the pitfalls of misdiagnosis, overtreatment, or undertreatment described in the preceding pages, these can be diminished. First, the concept of reality as depicted by television commercials must be corrected. It is simply not true that healthy reality is all blissful, that every discomfort constitutes a sickness, and that one therefore needs medication for every annoyance, particularly insomnia or being "edgy." It is important to realize that over-the-counter medications are chemically active substances that can have undesirable effects on the person, both physically and emotionally. While aspirin or an equivalent drug for a minor headache or a laxative taken *occasionally* are usually harmless, any medication that is taken frequently or regularly can cause trouble, and the symptom that requires frequent use of medication may indicate a condition that requires evaluation. If the sufferer is in doubt, a physician should be consulted about what is considered acceptable "occasionally."

Second, some unhealthy practices are so widespread that they are considered normal, and one is therefore not likely to implicate them as causative of symptoms. Many people do not consider alcohol harmful unless it is consumed in excessive quantities, but this is not true. What many people consider "moderate" or "social" drinking can be both physically and emotionally destructive. Alcohol can be toxic to many body tissues and can produce a variety of symptoms. Persons with either physical or emotional discomfort would be well-advised to completely eliminate the use of alcohol. If a person finds that he cannot eliminate alcohol for an extended period of time, even on a trial basis, he may indeed have an alcohol–dependency problem.

Similarly, if one's symptoms include anxiety manifestations, caffeine should be eliminated. People should also look at their dietary habits in general. Instruction on a balanced diet, with adequate vitamins and minerals, can be obtained by consultation with a competent dietician. All hospitals have dieticians on their staff, and arrangements can usually be made with a dietician for review of one's diet and for appropriate guidance.

Mind-altering drugs of whatever type, if not prescribed by a physician, should be completely curtailed. Even if the drugs are initially prescribed by a physician, one should have their value reconsidered by the physician. Going for psychological or psychiatric help while using a brain-affecting drug in addictive fashion is senseless. This is comparable to taking one's automobile in for a tune-up while one is periodically putting gravel into the carburetor. No mechanic, however excellent and competent, can be expected to restore the engine to smooth and efficient functioning if there is gravel in the carburetor; it is equally foolish to expect a psychiatrist or psychologist to help restore healthy emotional functioning while one is putting alcohol or other mind-altering drugs into the brain.

While modern medical technology has provided physicians with excellent diagnostic techniques, their very excellence has led some physicians to forget that the doctor himself can be the most sensitive and accurate diagnostic instrument. Some important aspects of a patient's being and functioning simply cannot be detected and recorded by any technological gadget. We were instructed in medical school that if a laboratory test conflicts with the doctor's clinical impression, it is most likely the laboratory that is in error rather than the physician. Flashing lights and computer printouts may indeed be impressive, but they must be subordinate to the physician. If people realize that the human is more than a bundle of complex chemicals, they will understand why physicians cannot be replaced by computers.

I am aware that some physicians, prior to their initial personal contact with the patient, will have the patient undergo a blood count, chemical profile, urinalysis, and perhaps several other studies. These laboratory tests may indeed be most helpful, but I believe they should not be performed until after the doctor has interviewed and examined the patient and has reached an initial clinical impression. Modern technology notwithstanding, the traditional history and physical must come first. Doctors should have an impression of the totality of the patients before analyzing their component parts.

Laboratory studies performed prior to the personal interview and examination can mislead physicians. An abnormal laboratory finding may skew the physicians' thinking, and their assumptions that they already know what is wrong with their patients may preclude their attentiveness to other factors that may be more significant in the patients' problems.

Above all, do not go around shopping from specialist to specialist until you have found someone who agrees to do what you want to have done. Unfortunately, a small minority of doctors are opportunists and exploit their profession, and given the legalities on restraint of trade and the fact that the state and not the medical society grants the license to practice medicine, legitimate medicine can do little to eliminate them. But by describing one's symptoms in a particular way, one may present a case for medical intervention by a completely reputable and ethical physician who may not have access to all the facts.

If you have a persistent severe pain problem, ask your primary physician for a referral to a comprehensive pain management center. Do not importune him for potent pain-killing medication, because this may ultimately result in an addiction problem superimposed upon the pain, and the latter would probably no longer be relieved by even potent medication.

It is understandable that when medical science cannot offer the desired relief, people may turn to any one that does hold out promise and hope. It is regrettable that some people exploit human suffering for their personal gain. Let your primary physician advise you on the use of any method that is not medically recognized as valuable.

If all medically accepted treatments have been exhausted and you wish to try a folk remedy or an equivalent that carries no risk, there may be no harm in this. However, some of these "cures" are not innocuous, and certainly none should be permitted to be substituted for treatment methods that have been demonstrated to be effective.

Getting back to emotional reactions, many distressing conditions may be normal, and their "treatment" may actually be harmful. The management of grief is a classic example. Mourning is indeed painful, yet this is the method whereby one adjusts to a loss and reorganizes one's personality to continue on with life. Smothering the grief process with tranquilizers may result in a delayed grief reaction, which can become a definite psychiatric problem. People who are in mourning need emotional support rather than emotional anesthesia.

Finally, as an interested citizen, you should become active in and supportive of mental health activities in your community. Historically, people with emotional problems have not been given priority in the allocation of human services. This negative attitude toward mental illness still prevails and is responsible for some health institutions diluting the quality of mental health care offered and for governmental funding agencies reducing financial support for these services. As pointed out, increasing mental health services by economizing on medical staff can lead to tragic misdiagnosis and inappropriate treatment. Prevention of such errors by an interested citizen group is not merely altruistic, because it can ultimately benefit oneself if the need arises.

Index